THYROID DISEASE AND MUSCLE DYSFUNCTION

THYROID DISEASE AND MUSCLE DYSFUNCTION

IAN RAMSAY

M.D.(Edin.), M.R.C.P.(Lond.), M.R.C.P.(Edin.)

Consultant Physician, Regional Endocrine Centre, North Middlesex Hospital, London, N.18

WILLIAM HEINEMANN MEDICAL BOOKS LTD.

First published 1974

ISBN 0 433 272 554

PRINTED IN ENGLAND BY
THE WHITEFRIARS PRESS LTD, LONDON AND TONBRIDGE

To Patty and Augustus
for their help

FOREWORD

Some ten years ago a young clinician, Ian Ramsay, came to my laboratory. He was well trained and had the critical attitude of the British school at its best. He was determined to study thyrotoxic myopathy by all available methods. In record time he acquainted himself thoroughly with quantitative electromyography. In the intervening years he has used this and other methods to study muscle dysfunction in a unique consecutive series of patients with thyrotoxicosis. His papers on the subject mark real advances in the understanding of metabolic muscle disease.

Two of Ramsay's findings are rare in muscle disease and impressed me as being of basic importance:

(i) Structural changes were mild or absent although weakness and wasting and electromyographic evidence of "fibre loss" were pronounced.

(ii) There was a remarkable return to normal of the electromyographic abnormalities and of weakness and wasting a few months after successful treatment of hyperthyroidism. These findings indicate transient block of muscle fibres rather than destruction and repair.

Muscle disorders in thyroid disease are a fascinating subject, bordering as they do on endocrinology, neurology, pathology and neurophysiology. Since Dr. Ramsay has been one of the pioneers in this area he is exceptionally qualified to present the state of knowledge, which he does from his own work and by a critical evaluation of the work of others.

It gives me pleasure to introduce his lucid account of muscle dysfunction in thyroid disease. The book fills a need.

Fritz Buchthal
Institute of Neurophysiology,
University of Copenhagen.

PREFACE

This book is written in an attempt to clarify one of those areas in medicine where specialities overlap, namely endocrinology and neurology, though many of the clinical problems to be considered are encountered by the general physician. In the last decade or so increasing attention has been drawn to the association between abnormalities of skeletal muscle and derangement of thyroid function. Thus thyrotoxic myopathy, previously thought to be rare, is now known to be common; muscular abnormalities are being more frequently described in patients with hypothyroidism; and the association of Myasthenia Gravis and Periodic Paralysis with hyperthyroidism is also well recognized. That there are these associations is not surprising considering that thyroid hormone plays a major part in regulating the production of energy in the body, and indeed it is to be hoped that investigation of these diseases will throw more light on the controlling mechanisms of muscle metabolism.

My thanks are due to the two thyrotoxic patients with severe myopathy who first stimulated my interest in the subject and to the Royal Victoria Hospital, Belfast, which generously supported my initial researches. I am also grateful to Miss G. Pentelow of King's College Hospital Medical School Library and her staff for helping to check the references.

I. R.

December 1973

ACKNOWLEDGEMENTS

Grateful acknowledgements are made to the following publishers for allowing their illustrations to be reproduced.

Chapter 1

Fig. 3: *The Lancet*
Figs. 4 and 7: The Clarendon Press, Oxford
Figs. 8, 9, 10 and 11: The Mayo Clinic Proceedings

Chapter 2

Figs. 3, 4 and 6: *Acta Neurologica Scandinavica*
Fig. 5: The Royal Australasian College of Physicians
Fig. 7: Archives of Neurology
Figs. 8 and 9: The Muscular Dystrophy Group of Great Britain

Chapter 3

Figs. 1 and 2: *The British Medical Journal*
Fig. 3: Neurology
Fig. 4: The American Medical Association
Figs. 5, 6, 7, 8, 9 and 10: *The Johns Hopkins Medical Journal*

Chapter 4

Fig. 2: Archives of Physical Medicine and Rehabilitation
Figs. 3, 4 and 5: Mayo Clinic Proceedings
Fig. 6: *Journal of Clinical Endocrinology and Metabolism*
Figs. 7, 8, 9, 10 and 12: American Medical Association
Fig. 11: Excerpta Medica Foundation
Figs. 13, 14, 15 and 16: *Journal of Cell Biology*

CONTENTS

CHAPTER 1

THYROTOXIC MYOPATHY

Severe muscular weakness and wasting occurring in patients with thyrotoxicosis has, comparatively recently, been regarded as rare (Whitfield and Hudson, 1961). The association however was first noticed by both Graves (1835) and Basedow (1840) in their descriptions of hyperthyroidism. Quite a long time elapsed after their observations before du Cazal in 1885 (Sattler, 1952) and Bathurst in 1895 specifically described patients who presented with severe muscular atrophy and weakness as the first indication of their thyrotoxicosis. Bathurst noticed the predominantly proximal involvement of the arms and legs and described how his patient found it difficult to rise from the lying or kneeling positions without using his arms.

Possibly because of the protean nature of thyrotoxic symptoms and signs and because of the ease with which florid hyperthyroidism can be diagnosed, the presence of myopathy was neglected and in the years between 1895 and 1962 only 73 cases could be found by Ramsay (1964) in the English, German and French literature.* Waldenström said in 1945 that thyrotoxic myopathy was extremely uncommon and Whitfield and Hudson (1961) thought that it was of considerable rarity. Without a doubt the severe form, presenting with myopathic symptoms which overshadow all else, is relatively uncommon, but recent work done in the last decade and a half suggests that these 73 published cases represent the visible top of the iceberg and that if thyrotoxic patients are carefully examined clinically and electromyographically, a majority will be found to have muscle involvement (Pipberger, Kälin and Wegmann, 1955;

* Bathurst (1895), Ayer, Means and Lerman (1934), Starling and Brain (1938), Darke, Hunt and Brain (1938), Parsons and Twort (1939), MacKenzie (1940), del Castillo, de la Balze and Caul (1940), Morgan and Williams (1940), McEachern and Ross (1942), Devic *et al.* (1942), Bartels and Pizer (1944), Thorn and Eder (1946), Froment, Gallavardin and Devic (1946), Devic *et al.* (1947), Sanderson and Adey (1949), Quinn and Worcester (1951), Zierler (1951), Sanderson and Adey (1952), Millikan and Haines (1953), Kite, McClintock and Graves (1954), Sacrez, Lausecker and Isch (1955), Hoffenburg and Eales (1956), Collings and Lienhard (1957), Boström and Hed (1958), Hed, Kirstein and Lundmark (1958), Melville (1959), Ellis and Carey (1961), Whitfield and Hudson (1961) and Havard (1962).

Hed, Kirstein and Lundmark, 1958; Gimlette, 1959; Havard *et al.*, 1963; Satoyoshi, Murakami and Torii, 1963; Ramsay, 1965, 1966).

Analysis of the literature on 73 patients with "chronic thyrotoxic myopathy" (Ramsay, 1964)

The age at presentation was the same for both sexes, with an average of 47·7 years. Normally in an unselected group of thyrotoxics one would expect at least a 3 : 1 female : male ratio, but 38 of the patients were male, making virtually a 1 : 1 ratio. The female patients had had symptoms of thyrotoxicosis for an average of 25·3 months and weakness for 22·5 months compared with 11·3 months and 11·1 months respectively for the men. It is interesting to note that the symptoms of myopathy were an early feature of the illness. The mean weight loss was rather similar in the two groups, being 16·6 kg for the males and 15·1 kg for the females, but of course this represents a greater percentage weight loss in the female sex and would accord with the much longer duration of their symptoms.

Although the patients were reported in the literature because of their myopathic features, in fact in only 23 % were they the presenting complaint. In most of the other patients the onset of muscular weakness was concurrent or followed shortly after the onset of the usual features of hyperthyroidism. The characteristic complaints were difficulty in climbing stairs, rising from a kneeling position or from a low chair, getting up out of bed, lifting the arms for such tasks as combing the hair, hanging curtains or putting things on shelves. Some patients experienced enormous fatigue while walking even on the level and a few noticed weakness of every muscle movement. There was no relationship between the muscle weakness and the presence or absence of exophthalmos or of ophthalmoplegia.

In 49·3 % of the patients the only muscles affected were the proximal muscles of the shoulder and pelvic girdles. In 34·3 % distal as well as proximal muscles were involved. In the remaining 16·4 % of the patients there was dysfunction of the bulbar muscles in addition to involvement of all skeletal muscles. There were no differences between the two sexes as to the groups of muscles affected by the myopathic process. Muscle pain, stiffness and contractions were noted in one patient by Hoffenburg and Eales (1956), cramps were described in two patients (Sanderson and Adey, 1952; Millikan and Haines, 1953) and were the presenting feature in a recent case (Araki, Terao, Matsumoto, Narazaki and Kuroiwa, 1968). Muscular aching was prominent in one of Whitfield and Hudson's (1961) patients.

In the patients with bulbar weakness, difficulty in speaking was the most prominent symptom. There was an inability to pronounce words properly, hoarseness or an alteration in the quality of the voice. Dysphagia was the second common problem and in one patient there was nasal regurgitation when swallowing fluids.

Spontaneous muscle movements were seen in 41·7% of the men with thyrotoxic myopathy, but in only 3·2% of the women. It is possible that this difference could be due to the preservation of a thicker layer of subcutaneous fat in women. The movements were variously described as being fasciculation or fibrillation, though the latter is rather a misnomer since strictly speaking it is an electromyographic phenomenon produced by the contraction of single muscle fibres and cannot be seen through the skin (Thomas, 1963). There is no clear explanation so far for these spontaneous muscle movements. Abnormally sensitive motor end plates were thought by some to be the cause of the phenomenon (McEachern and Ross, 1942; Kite, McLintock and Graves, 1954). Harman and Richardson (1954) thought that the movements were identical to the myokymia which may occur in normal people, especially when fatigued. Characteristically this is seen as coarse muscular twitching. It is not affected by spinal or high nerve block, is not made worse by prostigmine but is abolished by curare. Electromyographic studies show an increased excitability of nerve tissue.

Unselected thyrotoxic patients

The findings in the above group of patients, selected because of the prominence of their myopathy, can be compared with several series of unselected thyrotoxic patients (see Table 1.1). It can be seen that about 5% of all thyrotoxic patients have weakness as their presenting complaint, a third to a half have it as a symptom and 60 to 80% are weak on clinical examination. The type of weakness noted is similar to that described in the patients with chronic myopathy, namely difficulty in walking upstairs, rising out of a chair, brushing or combing the hair without resting, lifting things from high shelves, putting up curtains, playing the piano and carrying shopping baskets; some of the men who were engaged in manual labour noticed that they required help in lifting heavy objects which previously they could manage by themselves (Havard *et al.*, 1963; Ramsay, 1966). A few patients noticed aching in their muscles (Ramsay, 1964).

In Ramsay's series (1966) 63% of the patients had proximal muscle involvement alone. This was usually both weakness and

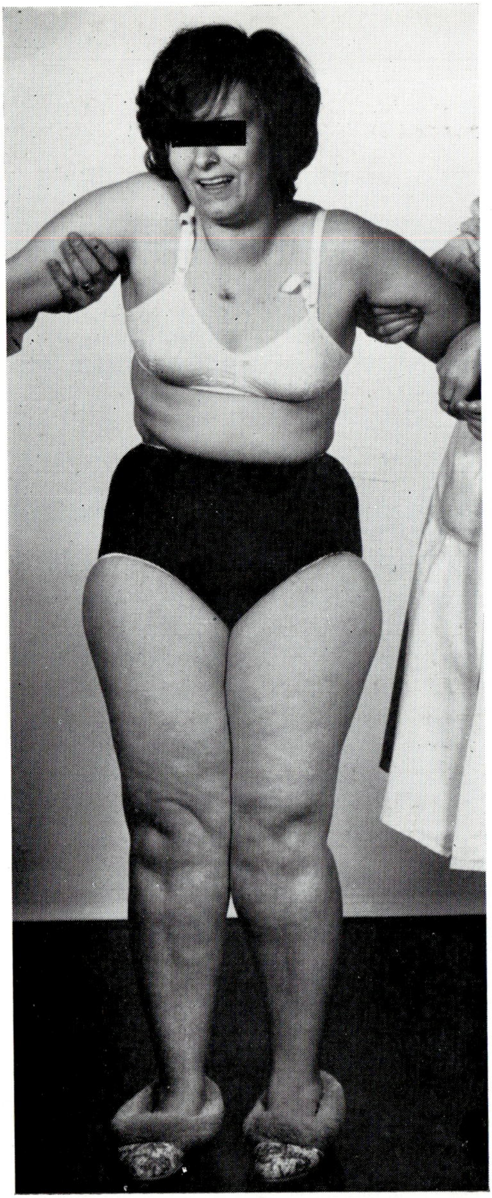

Figure 1.1. Female thyrotoxic patient with well preserved fat stores who had such a severe proximal myopathy that she was unable to stand unaided. (Patient of Dr. C. G. McKerron).

TABLE 1.1

A comparison of the symptoms and signs of weakness in 73 patients with chronic thyrotoxic myopathy and in several series of unselected thyrotoxic patients

Series	No. of patients	Weakness as the presenting complaint %	Weakness as a symptom %	Weakness clinically %
Recorded cases of myopathy (Ramsay, 1964)	73	23	100	100
Pipberger, Kälin and Wegmann (1955)	13		61·5	69·2
Gimlette (1959)	40		32·5	60
Havard *et al.* (1963)	50	6	34	80
Satoyoshi *et al.* (1963a)	240			61
Ramsay (1965, 1966)	54	3·7	50	81·5
Ludin, Spiess and Koenig (1969)	13	7·7	54	61·5

wasting though occasionally there was weakness without any obvious clinical atrophy. In only 2 patients out of 54 was there thought to be atrophy without any weakness. In a further 18·5% of the patients there was distal muscle involvement in the limbs in addition to proximal myopathy. In all, 81·5% of the unselected thyrotoxics had clinical evidence of a muscle disorder.

The frequency and distribution of myopathic change, were the same in both sexes. Muscle atrophy was easier to detect in men because of a smaller amount of subcutaneous fat. Fig. 1.1 shows a woman with gross myopathy who still has large fat stores. There was no significant differences between the ages of the patients who had myopathy and those who did not. This evidence suggests that muscle involvement in thyrotoxicosis affects both sexes and the elderly and young equally. The average age of the unselected thyrotoxic patients (47·9 years) was similar to that of the 73 patients with chronic myopathy described in the literature (47·7 years).

As has been noted already in the analysis of the 73 patients with chronic myopathy (Table 1.2), in Ramsay's series the muscular weakness came on shortly after the start of other thyrotoxic symptoms, suggesting that muscle dysfunction is an early feature of hyperthyroidism. Moreover there was no direct correlation with the severity of the thyrotoxicosis as measured by serum protein bound iodine or by the amount of weight lost.

Havard *et al.* (1963) noted obvious wasting of the shoulder or

TABLE 1.2

A comparison between 73 patients with chronic thyrotoxic myopathy and 54 unselected thyrotoxics (Ramsay, 1964)

	73 "chronic thyrotoxic myopathy" patients	54 unselected thyrotoxics
Mean age (years)	47·7	47·9
Male/female ratio	38:35	14:40
Mean duration of thyrotoxic symptoms (months)	18·5	6·6
Mean duration of weakness (months)	16·4	5·0
Mean weight loss (kg)	15·9	8·0
Ophthalmoplegia (%)	6·2	7·4
Muscles affected:		
Proximal alone (%)	49·3	63
Proximal and distal (%)	34·3	18·5
Generalized and bulbar (%)	16·4	0

pelvic girdle muscles in 46% of their patients. They quantified the reduction in muscle bulk by soft tissue radiographs and showed that there was an increase in size after the patient had been made euthyroid. In 80% of the patients there was muscle weakness. The muscles commonly involved were the deltoid, the supraspinatus and quadriceps. Winging of the scapulae because of weakness of serratus anterior was seen quite often and gluteal atrophy was prominent in many of the male patients. The frequency with which the various

TABLE 1.3

The frequency with which the various muscles were affected by weakness and/or atrophy (Ramsay, 1966)

	No. of patients		No. of patients
Supraspinatus	33	Serratus anterior	5
Triceps	33	Pectorals	4
Deltoid	30	Hypothenar muscles	4
Infraspinatus	28	Temporalis	3
Biceps brachialis	28	Flexors of wrist	3
Iliopsoas	26	Sternomastoid	2
Quadriceps	11	Biceps femoris	2
Glutei	9	Interossei	2
Extensors of wrist	6	Flexors of fingers	1
Thenar muscles	6		

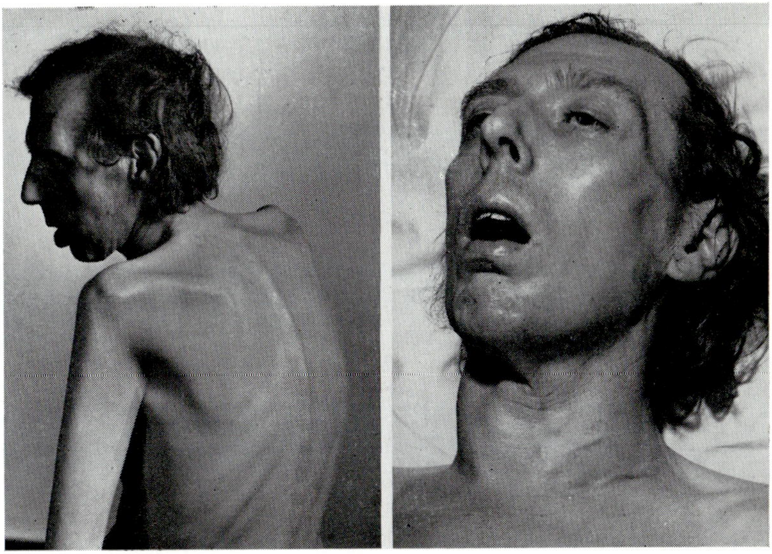

(*a*) (*b*)

Figure 1.2(*a*). Male thyrotoxic patient aged 45 showing wasting of the shoulder girdle muscles. (Patient of Dr. S. Oram).

Figure 1.2(*b*). Wasting of the temporal muscles.

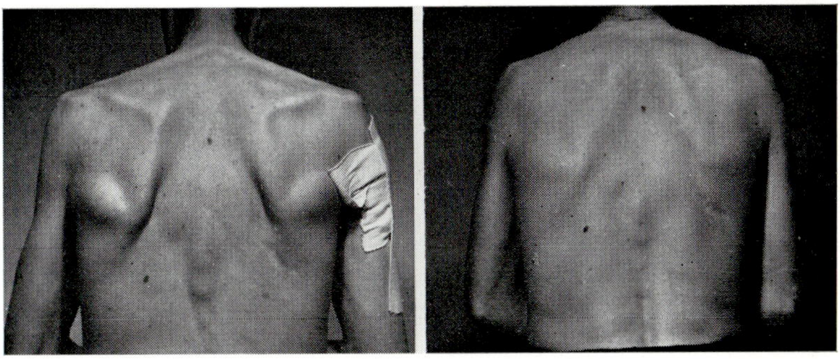

(*a*) (*b*)

Figure 1.3(*a*). Male, aged 38 showing marked wasting of the shoulder girdle muscles while thyrotoxic. (From Ramsay, 1966).

Figure 1.3(*b*). The same patient four months after becoming euthyroid.

muscles were involved in Ramsay's (1966) series can be seen in Table 1.3. Muscles of the shoulder girdle were more often involved than those of the pelvic girdle and extensor muscles were twice as commonly affected as flexor muscles. Figure 1.2(a) shows a patient with typical shoulder girdle wasting at the time of diagnosis of thyrotoxicosis. In Fig. 1.2(b) wasting of the temporalis muscle can also be seen. Figure 1.3 shows the return of muscle bulk in another patient four months after he had become euthyroid. No patients in Ramsay's (1966) series had distal muscle involvement without proximal myopathy. Exactly the same situation has been noted in the published cases of chronic myopathy, except that more of the patients had distal muscle involvement (see Table 1.2) and, in addition, 16·4% had evidence of bulbar paresis.

Recently Joasoo, Murray and Steinbeck (1970) described 12 cases of thyrotoxic myopathy, 10 of them seen over a two-year period, in whom bulbar muscles were involved. Eight of the patients were women and four were men. Their ages ranged from 21 to 74 years and clinically all were suffering from a proximal myopathy. In addition, six of the 12 had evidence of a distal myopathy, though, if electromyography of the distal muscles had been done, it is likely that the proportion would have been higher, since Ramsay (1965) found electromyographic evidence of a myopathy in distal muscles 2·5 times as frequently as clinical examination would suggest. Dysphagia was the commonest symptom of their bulbar myopathy and was just as bad for liquids as for solids. In a number of cases liquids were passed into the nose during swallowing attempts. Changes in the voice were common and consisted of a nasal quality, weakness of word production or hoarseness. Many of the patients had a myopathic facies and three of the patients had difficulty in chewing. Generally speaking there seems to be a decreasing order of susceptibility of the different muscle groups to the thyrotoxic process, the proximal muscles being affected first, then distal muscles and finally bulbar muscles. There is also some evidence to suggest that respiratory muscles are weak in thyrotoxicosis (Massey *et al.*, 1967).

The tendon reflexes tend to be normal or brisk in hyperthyroidism (Ramsay, 1966; Ludin *et al.*, 1969), but accurate measurement of the duration of the Achilles reflex shows that it is nearly always diminished (Lawson, 1958; Abraham, Atkinson and Roscoe, 1966).

Prostigmine or edrophonium (Tensilon) was given to 27 of the cases of chronic myopathy described in the literature. No increase in power was detected in 24 cases. It produced a good response in only one patient (McEachern and Ross, 1942) and a slight response in another two (Sanderson and Adey, 1949; Melville, 1959). Havard *et al.* (1963) tested muscle strength in 49 thyrotoxics before and and 30 minutes after 1·5 mg of intramuscular neostigmine. Forty-three patients showed no increase in power though 6 were thought to be stronger. Osserman and Silver (1961) found neostigmine to be ineffective in thyrotoxics. Ramsay (1966) could demonstrate no significant difference in the length of time for which thyrotoxic subjects could maintain their legs at an angle of 45 degrees to the horizontal before and after the intravenous injection of edrophonium chloride.

Electromyography

The first reports of electromyographic abnormalities in chronic thyrotoxic myopathy were made by Sanderson and Adey (1949, 1952) who described a significant reduction in mean action potential duration, low action potential voltage and an increase in the number of polyphasic potentials. Millikan and Haines (1953) found normal electromyograms (E.M.Gs.), though since their report Boström and Hed (1958), Hed, Kirstein and Lundmark (1958), Whitfield and Hudson (1961) and Havard (1962) have all reported E.M.G. patterns which were typical of myopathy in their patients with clinical involvement of muscle.

Since 1955 nine series of thyrotoxic patients have been studied electromyographically and the results are summarized in Table 1.4. The earlier published papers have given qualitative estimations of E.M.G. findings and any difference in the results so obtained could be due to observer error. Others (Yates, 1963; Ramsay, 1965; Vilppula and Buchthal, 1970) used a quantitative method in which 20 to 27 different areas in each muscle were sampled and the mean action potential duration was compared to the normal for that patient's age. Allowing for the small number of patients studied in some of the series, the findings are remarkably similar in their demonstration of electromyographic abnormalities in a majority of thyrotoxic patients. In Ramsay's (1965) series just over 90% of the patients were found to have evidence of myopathy in their proximal muscles and 43% in their distal muscles. Figure 1.4(a) shows the shortened mean action potential duration in the deltoid muscle of thyrotoxic patients compared to controls and Fig. 1.4(b) shows the return towards normality on re-testing four months after the patients had become euthyroid. Figure 1.5 shows the less common E.M.G. changes in a distal muscle. This tendency for less frequent involve-

TABLE 1.4

Reports of electromyograms (E.M.G.s) done on thyrotoxic patients

	No. of patients	EMG evidence of myopathy %	Characteristic EMG features
Pipberger *et al.* (1955)	13	92·3	Shortening of action potentials, increase in polyphasicity, decrease in amplitude. Normal interference pattern.
Hed *et al.* (1958)	17	100	In areas sampled 75–100% of potentials were of short duration or polyphasic. "Dense" or "scanty" interference pattern.
Gimlette (1959)	40		"Myopathic" pattern in the majority.
Havard *et al.* (1963)	50	88	Motor units either polyphasic or shorter than normal.
Satoyoshi *et al.* (1963a, b)	39	61·5	Unspecified.
Yates (1963, 1965)	10	70	Shortened action potential duration.
Ramsay (1965)	54	92·6	Statistically significant reduction in action potential duration and increase in percentage polyphasicity.
Ludin *et al.* (1969)	13	77	Shortening of mean action potential duration and increase in polyphasic potentials.
Vilppula and Buchthal (1970)	13	84·6	Reduction in action potential duration and increased polyphasic potentials.

ment of the distal muscles has also been noted by Pipberger, Kälin and Wegmann (1955). The thyrotoxics had a slightly higher percentage of polyphasic potentials than the controls, with again a return to normality after treatment had been effective. Havard *et al.* (1963) and Yates (1965) have also noted normal E.M.G.s in their patients following clinical recovery.

A reduced mean action potential, measured on minimal effort, signifies the presence of a primary muscle disease and it is not specific for thyrotoxicosis (Kugelberg, 1947, 1949; Pinelli and Buchthal, 1953; Buchthal and Pinelli, 1953; Eaton and Lambert, 1957). It has not been found in patients with disuse atrophy resulting from up to six months of immobilization (Buchthal, 1957).

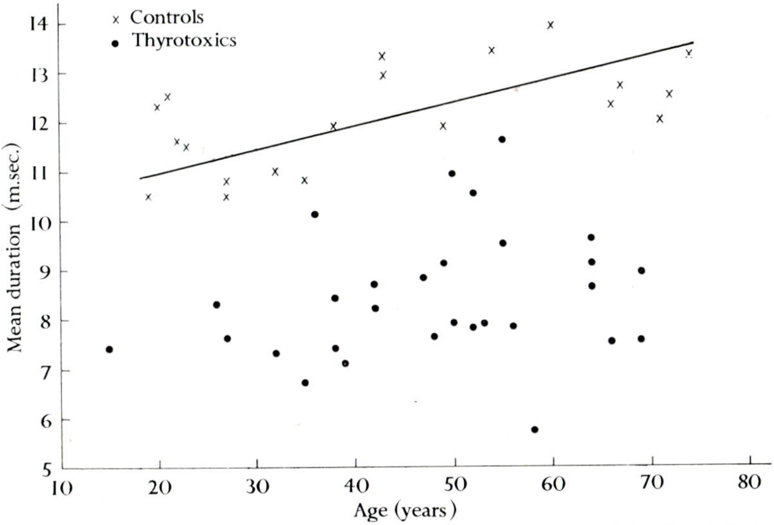

Figure 1.4(a). Showing the reduced mean action potential in the deltoid muscles of thyrotoxic patients compared with controls. Note the normal increase in mean action potential duration with age. (From Ramsay, 1965).

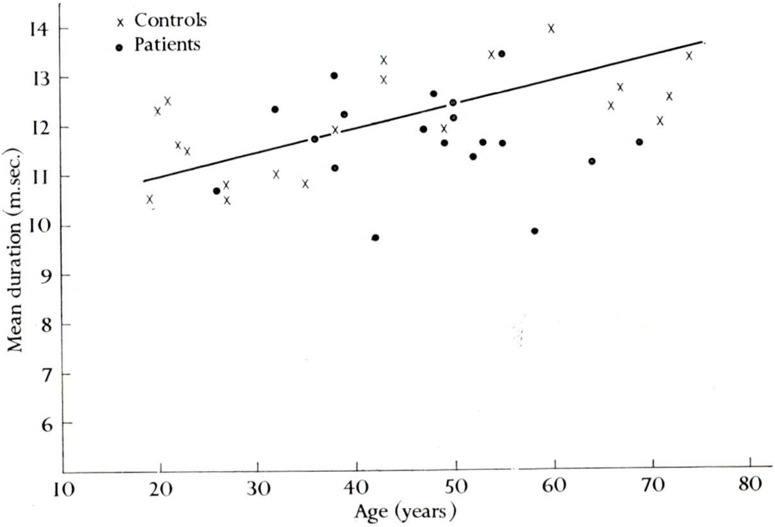

Figure 1.4(b). Mean action potential durations in the same patients four months after they had become euthyroid. (From Ramsay, 1965).

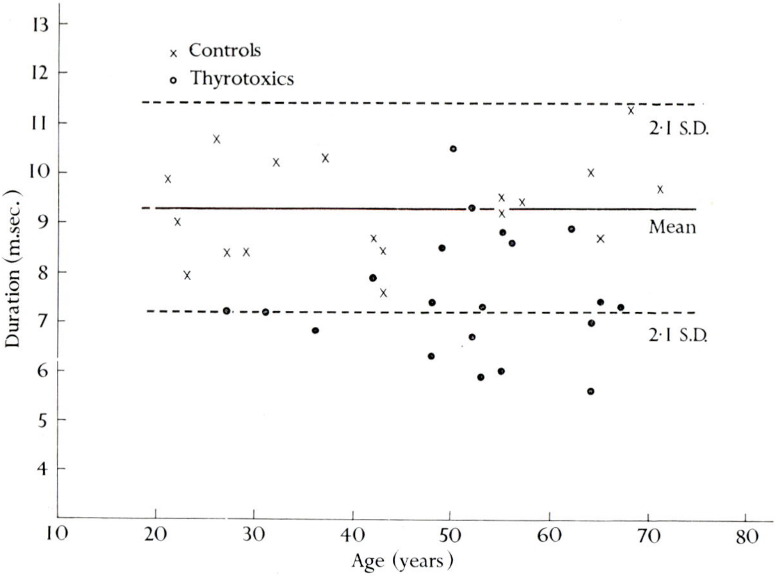

Figure 1.5. Showing the reduced mean action potential duration in a distal muscle (abductor digiti quinti) of only 43% of thyrotoxic patients. Note that there is no increase in mean action potential duration with age in control subjects. (From Ramsay, 1965).

The voltage of the potentials recorded at minimal effort was generally reduced (Ramsay, 1965), but a statistical analysis did not reveal that they were lower than the control values. Buchthal (1957) has pointed out that the mean amplitude must deviate from the normal by more than 50% in order to become significant. A reduction in the peak-to-peak voltage of the interference pattern taken during maximal effort has been found in myopathies in general (Kugelberg, 1947, 1949) and in thyrotoxicosis in particular (Hed, Kirstein and Lundmark, 1958), though statistically it is not such a good criterion for the diagnosis of a myopathy as the estimation of the mean action potential duration (Ramsay, 1965).

Spontaneous E.M.G. activity, in the form of fibrillation potentials and fasciculation has been rarely seen in thyrotoxicosis, though it was relatively more common in distal muscles than in proximal (Pipberger, Kälin and Wegmann, 1955; Hed, Kirstein and Lundmark, 1958; Havard *et al.*, 1963; Ramsay, 1965; Ludin, Spiess and Koenig, 1969). Though the two patients with fibrillation potentials reported by Hed, Kirstein and Lundmark (1958) probably had a lower motor neurone lesion, the presence of fibrillation does not necessarily indicate denervation (Eaton and Lambert, 1957) and it has been shown by Adrian and Gelfan (1933) that fibrillation can result from ionic differences across the muscle fibre membrane.

Recently however Ludin and his colleagues (1969) have raised the question as to whether the E.M.G. changes in distal muscles in thyrotoxics might not be evidence of a neuropathy rather than a myopathy. Unlike Ramsay (1965) who found clear evidence of a myopathy, with reduced mean action duration and increased polyphasisity in a distal muscle of the upper limb (abductor digiti quinti), Ludin, Spiess and Koenig (1969) investigated the small muscles of the foot. They diagnosed neuropathy if any two of the following three criteria were met: loss of motor units at maximal voluntary effort, fibrillation potentials or positive sharp waves at rest in at least two places and increase of the mean action potential duration. Of their 13 patients 6 had a reduced interference pattern at full voluntary effort, whereas all of Ramsay's (1965) patients with other E.M.G. evidence of a distal myopathy had normal interference patterns. Ludin, Spiess and Koenig (1969) found fibrillation potentials and/or positive sharp waves in two to four places in the foot muscles of 5 patients (30%). Ramsay (1965) on the other hand found isolated fibrillation in only 3 out of 21 thyrotoxic patients whose abductor digiti quinti was sampled. Buchthal (1970) has commented that interpretation of the significance of fibrillation potentials and positive sharp waves can be difficult as they may occur in the genetic or acquired myopathies as well as in neuropathies. Ludin, Spiess and Koenig (1969) did find an increase in the mean action potential duration in 5 of their patients, which was in favour of a neuropathy, yet all motor nerve conduction velocities and distal latency times were normal in the patients with "neuropathic" distal E.M.Gs., as were orthodromic sensory conduction times in the distal part of the ulnar nerve. Moreover, the sensory nerve action potentials had a normal shape and amplitude, which is evidence against axonal degeneration. If a clinically significant neuropathy were present one would have expected there to be some changes in nerve conduction. However, demyelination in terminal nerve branches in one case of thyrotoxicosis (Hed, Kirstein and Lundmark, 1958) and swelling of the terminal axons and clubbing of the motor end plates in 27 out of 35 biopsies of the vastus medialis (Havard *et al.*, 1963) have been described and therefore the question of a neuropathy in thyrotoxicosis remains an open one.

Havard *et al.* (1963) found that there was a reasonable correlation

TABLE 1.5

Showing the increasing severity of E.M.G. changes related to the clinical extent of the myopathy in thyrotoxicosis (Ramsay, 1965)

Clinical assessment	Proximal muscle Deviation of MAPD* from predicted
No obvious myopathy	$2{\cdot}8 \pm 1{\cdot}2$ m sec.
(n = 10)	
Proximal myopathy	$3{\cdot}9 \pm 2{\cdot}6$ m sec.
(n = 34)	$(0{\cdot}05 > p > 0{\cdot}025)$
Proximal and distal myopathy	$4{\cdot}2 \pm 1{\cdot}3$ m sec.
(n = 10)	$(0{\cdot}02 > p > 0{\cdot}01)$

* Mean action potential duration.

between the degree of clinical weakness of their thyrotoxic patients and the severity of the electromyographic changes. Ramsay (1965), using the degree of E.M.G. change compared with the extent of the muscular involvement, showed (Table 1.5) that there was a significant difference between those patients who had proximal involvement and those who had none. Moreover, there was an even greater difference between these patients who had weakness and atrophy of the distal as well as the proximal muscles compared with those who had no muscle involvement.

No correlation has been shown between the severity of the E.M.G. findings and the degree of thyrotoxicosis (as measured by the clinical indices of Crooks, Murray and Wayne (1959) or the protein bound iodine values), the amount of weight lost or the duration of thyrotoxicosis (Havard *et al.*, 1963; Ramsay, 1965). There was no difference in the E.M.G. changes between male and female patients (Ramsay, 1965).

There is still no completely adequate explanation of the factors which determine the action potential duration in myopathies. Buchthal and Rosenfalck (1955) pointed out that in normal muscle the longer duration of the motor unit potential compared with that of the individual fibre was due to a temporal dispersion in the summation of the fibres of the motor unit and they suggested that differences in temporal dispersion could be explained by variations in the size of the end-plate region. The short durations recorded in muscles such as the abductor digiti quinti, compared with biceps brachii (Sacco, Buchthal and Rosenfalck, 1962) could probably be explained on this basis. Sacco and his colleagues postulated that the progressive increase in duration of the action potential after the age of 20 in most muscles (see Fig. 1.4) was due to a decrease in muscle volume with advancing years, leading to a closer crowding together of muscle fibres. This would cause the voltage of the initial and terminal components of the motor unit potential, normally picked up from fibres of sub-units lying more than 0·5 mm from the electrode, to be greater and thus more easily recorded. However, they were unable to explain why this increase in duration with age did not occur in the abductor digiti quinti (Fig. 1.5).

The shorter action potential duration in myopathies has been attributed to a decrease in the number of fibres in each sub-unit (Buchthal and Rosenfalck, 1963) which would render those potentials emanating from distant sub-units undetectable to the recording electrode. Since, in Ramsay's (1965) study, there was initially a reduction in action potential duration, with a restoration to normal levels once the patient had become euthyroid, it seems likely that the myopathy in thyrotoxicosis is due to a reversible decrease in functioning muscle fibres. This theory would also explain the increase in thyrotoxic muscle of polyphasic potentials on E.M.G., because a motor unit which, in a healthy person gives rise to a long action potential duration, owing to the large temporal dispersion of sub-unit potentials, would be expected to show a polyphasic outline if the number of fibres in each sub-unit was reduced in an irregular fashion (Buchthal and Rosenfalck, 1963). There may be other contributing factors, such as the finding by Coërs and Woolf (1959) of sprouting of terminal nerve-fibres in thyrotoxic myopathy. This could give rise to a raised incidence of polyphasic potentials by causing greater temporal dispersion as the result of slower conduction through immature nerve-fibres (Buchthal and Rosenfalck, 1963).

No abnormalities of nerve conduction in thyrotoxicosis were found by Ramsay (1965) or Ludin and his colleagues (1969), but Norris (1966) has reported abnormal facilitation of neuromuscular transmission during repetitive nerve stimulation at fast rates in an 81-year-old man. The changes were the same as those described in oat cell carcinoma of the bronchus, but the patient was alive and well a year later, after treatment of his hyperthyroidism and his neuromuscular transmission had returned to normal. Demyelinization and vacuolization of minor nerves (Hed, Kirstein and Lundmark, 1958), clubbing of the motor end plate and marked swellings of the terminal axons (Havard *et al.*, 1963) have been described histologically. However, the experimental studies of Zaimis and her colleagues (1965), done on thyroxine treated cats suggest that thyroid hormone does not act on the neuromuscular junction but rather on the muscle fibre itself.

Achilles tendon reflex time

Measurements of the velocity of the Achilles tendon jerks were first measured in thyroid disease by Chaney (1924). The first observations in hyperthyroidism were by Lambert *et al.* (1951) whose findings are summarized in Table 1.6. Although the mean duration of the time from the tap to the half relaxation time was significantly reduced compared with normals, they pointed out that more than 75% of the thyrotoxic patients had values which lay within the normal range. This obviously limits ankle jerk measurements as a diagnostic aid, but it does indicate that there is some alteration in the contractile mechanism of muscle in hyperthyroidism because nerve conduction is normal in thyrotoxicosis (Ramsay, 1965; Ludin, Spiess and Koenig, 1969). Since these observations many others have been made on Achilles reflex times by different authors, using different methods of measurement, which bedevils comparison, but in general the results are similar (Lawson, 1958; Gilson, 1959; Sharpe, 1961; Nuttall and Doe, 1964; Ringqvist, 1970). The Achilles reflex time however is constant for any given patient whose thyroid status remains unaltered, and the test is therefore of value in observing the changes brought about by treatment (Lawson and Weissbein, 1959). It should be noted that β adrenergic blockade by propranolol, a drug frequently used to alleviate some of the symptoms of thyrotoxicosis, but which has no effect on thyroid function, can significantly prolong the reflex time (Waal-Manning, 1969).

TABLE 1.6

Data from Lambert et al. (*1951*) *showing the reduction in the ankle jerk duration in thyrotoxic subjects compared to controls*

	Normals	Thyrotoxics	Significance
Tap to half relaxation time	mean 0·34 sec. Range 0·21–0·45 sec.	mean 0·26 sec. Range 0·18–0·35 sec.	$P < 0{\cdot}001$

Biochemistry

Apart from the usual indices of hyperthyroidism there have been no constant biochemical features either in patients reported as having myopathy or in unselected thyrotoxics. Generally speaking serum calcium levels are normal. Among a consecutive series of 49 thyrotoxic patients (Ramsay, 1964) the mean value was 10·0 mg and 40 patients were within the normal limits of 9·5–10·5 mg %. Three patients had calcium levels between 9·0 and 9·5 mg %, and 6 others were mildly hypercalcaemic, the highest figure being 11·9 mg %. Mean potassium levels were 4·3 m Eq/l, though 3 patients were just below the lower limit of normal (3·5 m Eq/l). Occasionally patients with severe thyrotoxic myopathy have been described with marked reduction in potassium levels (Collings and Wendell, 1957; Sanghvi *et al.*, 1959; Logothetis and Warner, 1962). In the case of the patient of Collings and Wendell (1957) the administration of potassium lessened the muscular weakness, but permanent relief was only obtained after the successful treatment of the thyrotoxicosis.

Muscle potassium and sodium

Several groups of workers have shown that there is a diminution of total exchangeable potassium (K^e) in thyrotoxicosis, with an increase after treatment (Munro, Renschler and Wilson, 1958; Staffurth, 1962; Shizume *et al.*, 1966). Wayne (1960) found that K^e was normal in thyrotoxics when related to lean-body mass rather than to total body weight and he thought that the decrease in K^e in patients was due to the diminution in lean-body mass which occurs in thyrotoxicosis. However, Jungers and Savoie (1963), comparing the results of K^e estimations in patients with hyperthyroidism with those for patients with anorexia nervosa, found that while both groups had lost the same amount of weight, there was a proportionately greater loss of potassium in the thyrotoxic patients. Shizume *et al.* (1966) demonstrated a significant reduction in K^e in thyrotoxics no matter whether it was related to body weight or to lean-body mass. An examination of Staffurth's (1962) figures show that the increase in K^e after treatment is relatively greater than the weight gain. In male patients the K^e increased by 46·2% after treatment, while the weight rose by 18% and the total body water by only 5·5%. An increase in extracellular water has been found in hyperthyroidism by Cachera *et al.* (1949a and b), as in other wasting diseases. Satoyoshi *et al.* (1963a) showed that there was a decrease in muscle cell water. Since the calculation of the lean-body mass depends upon estimations of total body water (Pace and Rathbun, 1945) it could well be that relating the K^e to this is subject to the same errors as that relating it to body weight for the double reason that the percentage of total water in the lean-body mass is disturbed in pathological states and the division of fluids between intra- and extracellular fluids is unknown in any given patient.

Direct measurement of muscle cell potassium has been made by Satoyshi and his colleagues (1963a). They found a significant reduction in intracellular potassium whether the values were calculated on a wet or dry weight basis or related to its concentration in intracellular water. A strong correlation was shown between dynamometric measurement of muscle power and intracellular potassium determinations. Other workers have denied a decrease in muscle cell potassium (Staffurth and Thompson, 1965) and at the moment the matter is not resolved (Shishiba *et al.*, 1966).

Muscle sodium concentrations were doubled in thyrotoxic muscle in the study of Satoyoshi *et al.* (1963a). Shizume and his colleagues (1966) also demonstrated a significant increase in total exchangeable body sodium whether related to body weight or lean-body mass. Liu and Overman (1964) have found an increase in intracellular sodium in thyroxine treated rats.

Creatine and creatinine metabolism

Creatine is synthesized in the liver from glycocyamine which originates in the kidneys. It is then taken up by the muscles and converted by phosphocreatine kinase into phosphocreatine. Phosphocreatine is necessary for muscle contraction, its probable role being in the immediate resynthesis of adenosine triphosphate (ATP) by the transfer of a phosphoryl group to adenosine diphosphate. Satoyoshi and his co-workers (1963a, b) found significantly reduced muscle creatine, phosphocreatine and ATP in thyrotoxics and showed that there was a correlation between muscle ATP concentrations and muscular strength. Phosphocreatine in muscle may be lowered because of the inhibiting effect of thyroxine on phosphocreatine kinase (Askonas, 1951) or because a normal intracellular potassium may be necessary for its formation (Grob, Liljestrand and Johns, 1957).

It is likely that creatine is unable to gain entry to thyrotoxic muscle (Thorn and Eder, 1946). The serum level therefore rises (Kuhlbäck, 1957; Satoyoshi *et al.*, 1963a), the renal threshold is exceeded and urinary excretion increases. This is the reason why thyrotoxic patients have a reduced tolerance to ingested creatine (Thorn and Eder, 1946; Wilkins and Fleischmann, 1946). Urinary creatine is lower in normal adult males than in females, with an upper limit of 150 mg per day (Wilder and Morgulis, 1953). The upper limit of normal for women is 200 mg per day (Wang, 1939). In thyrotoxicosis with and without obvious myopathy the excretion is generally raised, though the high levels in serum and urine may be reduced, usually within a day, by the administration of potassium chloride (Satoyoshi *et al.*, 1963a).

Creatine is broken down to creatinine by anhydration, so, since the amount of creatine in muscle is diminished, it is not surprising that the amount of creatinine found in the urine of hyperthyroid patients is usually reduced. It must be emphasized, however, that the increased urinary excretion of creatine and the diminished excretion of creatinine are not specific for thyrotoxicosis, but occur in other sorts of muscular dystrophies and myopathies and are found in normal old age (Zierler, 1951). Moreover, in some patients with thyrotoxic myopathy there was no significant creatinuria (Zierler, 1951). This has been explained by Hoch (1962) as being due to a failure of synthesis. The formation of creatine in the liver requires the presence of ATP for the transfer of a methyl group from methionine to glycocyamine (Kühlback, 1957).

In most patients given medical therapy there is a prompt early improvement in creatine tolerance suggesting that the inability of thyrotoxic muscle to take up creatine is a direct effect of excess thyroid hormone and is not entirely due to a reduced muscle mass. Creatine tolerance reverted to normal in all patients treated by thyroidectomy (Peters *et al.*, 1951).

Calcium and magnesium metabolism

There is very little information available about calcium and magnesium metabolism in thyrotoxicosis. As has been noted already (p. 17) serum calcium levels may sometimes be elevated in thyrotoxic patients. Although Kleeman and his colleagues (1958) found no difference between serum magnesium concentrations of thyrotoxics and those of controls, Kobayashi and Takeuchi (1967) found low levels in hyperthyroid patients which increased after treatment, and Neguib (1963) has claimed that thyrotoxic patients have shown an increase in muscular strength after treatment with magnesium chloride. Namikawa (1970) demonstrated a clear increase of calcium and magnesium in the muscle of thyrotoxic patients and there was a close correlation with PBl, I^{131} uptake, cholesterol and B.M.R. Similar abnormalities of a milder nature were found in experimental thyrotoxicosis. The work of Del Castillo and Katz (1954a, b) and of Jenkinson (1957) suggests that a calcium compound (Ca X) controls the nerve impulse induced release of acetylcholine and that more acetylcholine is released if the concentration of calcium is raised or that of magnesium lowered. It is possible that calcium and magnesium ions compete for the same receptor site or for the carrier molecule X. Theoretically, therefore, in thyrotoxicosis, there might be a variable interference in the release of acetylcholine according to the relative elevations in the concentrations of calcium and magnesium in muscle end-plates. It may also provide an explanation for the variable effect of thyrotoxicosis on patients with myasthenia gravis.

It has been shown by Margreth and his colleagues (Margreth, Salviati and Mussini, 1970) that there is a four-fold difference in the initial rate of calcium uptake by microsomes isolated from fast, white (Type II) muscles of rabbits compared with those of slow, red (Type I) muscles. They felt that the differing rates of accumulation of calcium in the sarcoplasmic reticulum played a part in the time scale of the contraction–relaxation cycle in fast muscle compared with slow. No information is yet available about any difference in rate of calcium uptake in proximal and distal muscles of thyrotoxic patients, which may have different proportions of Type I and Type II fibres (see p. 30), but the increased amount of calcium found in thyrotoxic muscle generally might provide a partial explanation for the faster twitch times and brisker tendon jerks found in hyperthyroidism.

Pyridoxine

The relationship between thyrotoxicosis and an impaired tryptophane tolerance test was first noted by Wachstein and Lobel in 1956. That this was caused by pyridoxine deficiency was confirmed by Wohl and his colleagues (1960). However the muscular weakness of hyperthyroidism was only helped by the administration of pyridoxine in one out of 14 patients in the series of Wohl *et al.* (1960) though there have been two other isolated reports of improvement (Rosenbaum, Portis and Soskin, 1941; Hamfelt and Wetterberg, 1964).

Muscle enzymes

Serum creatine phosphokinase (or, more properly, phosphocreatine kinase) has been reported to be normal in several small groups of thyrotoxic patients (Hess *et al.*, 1964; Pearce, Pennington and Walton, 1964; Griffiths, 1965; Ekbom *et al.*, 1966) or to be raised (Satoyoshi *et al.*, 1963a). However, in a large study which included 25 thyrotoxic patients, Graig and Smith (1965) were able to show that hyperthyroid patients had a significantly reduced level of serum creatine phosphokinase (CPK) compared with normal controls and euthyroid patients. There appeared to be an inverse relationship between the CPK and the PBI. This would fit in with the findings of Askonas (1951) that excess thyroxine has an inhibiting effect on the enzyme.

Satoyoshi *et al.* (1963a) found decreased aldolase, lactic dehydrogenase and total thiamine in thyrotoxic muscle but normal amounts in serum. However, the concentrations of free thiamine were normal in thyrotoxic muscle and serum, as was glutamic oxalocetic transaminase. The concentrations of creatine phosphokinase were lower in thyrotoxic muscle than in control tissue.

Elevation of serum malic dehydrogenase has been described in hyperthyroid Graves disease (Lieberthal, Benson and Klitgaard, 1963), as has serum ribonuclease (Leeper, 1963).

So far it has not been possible to explain all these enzyme changes on the basis of one action of thyroid hormone.

Steroid hormone metabolism in thyrotoxicosis

It has been noted (p. 2) that more male cases of chronic thyrotoxic myopathy have been found in the literature than female. Thus, one might speculate that there is some alteration in the production of the hormones which are known to affect skeletal muscle. Although cortisol synthesis is increased in thyrotoxicosis, this probably due to the fact that there is an accelerated clearance of cortisol by the liver (Peterson, 1958). Urinary 17-ketosteroids are low in hyperthyroidism (Engstrom and Mason, 1944; Peterson, 1958), and many men with chronic thyrotoxic myopathy have been noted to have testicular atrophy or azoospermia (Quinn and Worcester, 1951; Thorn and Eder, 1946; Asper and Wilson, 1957). It could therefore be surmised that thyrotoxic men with low 17-ketosteroids may lose a protein anabolic effect. However, in a survey of unselected thyrotoxics, Ramsay (1964) was unable to find any differences between the two sexes so far as the incidence of muscle weakness and electromyographic changes were concerned.

Muscle pathology

Askanazy (1898) was the first to describe changes in the muscles of thyrotoxic patients. He made an exhaustive study of four patients at post-mortem and found diffuse changes in all striated muscles, including the extrinsic muscles of the eye. There was infiltration of fat between the muscle fibres, atrophy of muscle fibres with a decrease in their diameter, proliferation and degeneration of muscle nuclei, loss of striations and vacuolization (Fig. 1.6). Cardiac and smooth muscle were not involved, nor were the abnormalities found in the

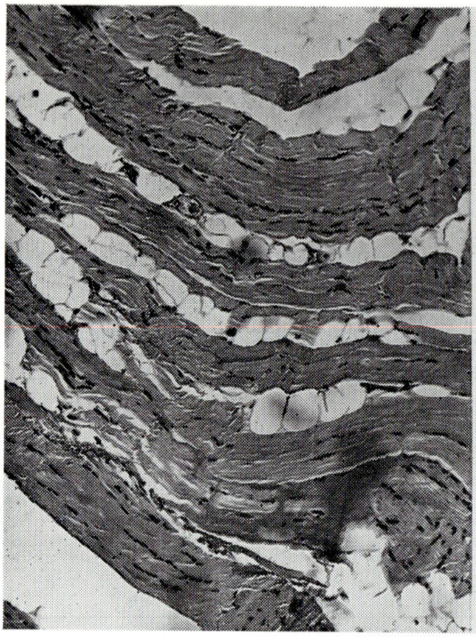

(*a*)

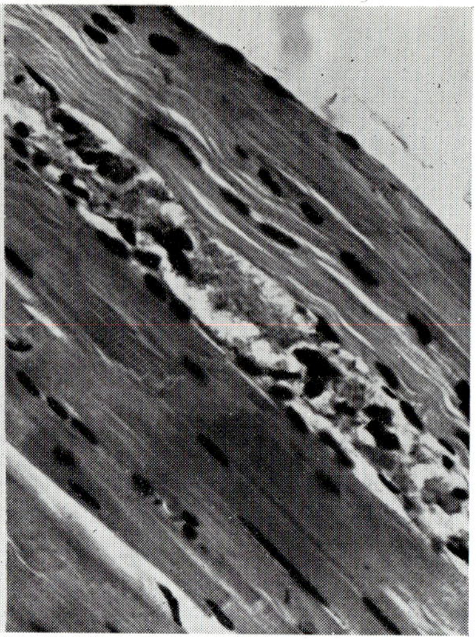

(*b*)

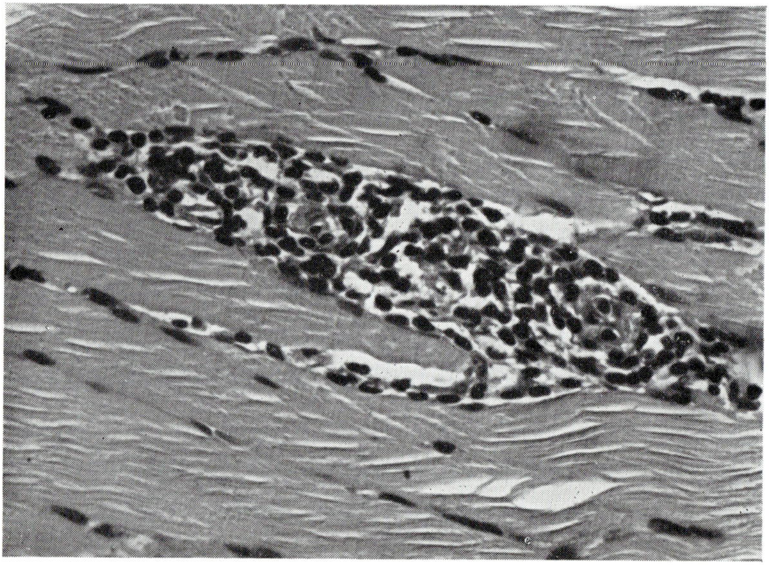

(*c*)

Figure 1.6. Abnormal histological appearances of skeletal muscle in thyrotoxicosis.

Figure 1.6(*a*). Infiltration of fat between the muscle fibres. (Van Gieson ×75).

Figure 1.6(*b*). Degenerating muscle fibre infiltrated with macrophages. (H & E, ×475).

Figure 1.6(*c*). Perivascular lymphorrhage (H & E, ×475).

same muscles in different patients. Since 1898 more reports have appeared. Many described much the same findings as Askanazy (Dudgeon and Urquhart, 1926; Morgan and Williams, 1940; Bartels and Pizer, 1944; Quinn and Worcester, 1951; Boström and Hed, 1958; Havard, 1962; Satoyoshi *et al.*, 1963a, b; Ramsay, 1964), but in addition aggregations of lymphocytes, or lymphorrhages (Fig. 1.6(c)), have been noted (Dudgeon and Urquhart, 1926; Liechti, 1938; Thorn and Eder, 1946; Hed, Kirstein and Lundmark, 1958; Whitfield and Hudson, 1961; Ramsay, 1964). Not infrequently, there have been no abnormal histological findings in patients with thyrotoxic myopathy (Morgan and Williams, 1940; Sanderson and Adey, 1949; Millikan and Haines, 1953; Kite, McLintock and Graves, 1954; Collings and Lienhard, 1957) and muscle degeneration (Fig. 1.6(b)) was not found in a recent series of thyrotoxic patients by Havard *et al.* (1963). However, some abnormalities were found in 23·3% of cases by Ramsay (1966) and in 68% of the patients of Satoyoshi and his co-workers (1963a). The latter authors found that when thyrotoxic symptoms were present for less than a year, abnormalities were present in 50% of cases, but rose to 85% if the patients had been ill for longer than one year. The smaller percentage in Ramsay's (1966) series can probably be explained by the shorter duration of thyrotoxic symptoms before presentation (mean 6·6 months). In neither series was there any correlation between the muscle biopsy findings and the severity of the thyrotoxicosis.

Ramsay (1966) found a constant reduction in mean muscle fibre diameter in thyrotoxic patients, the average being 12 μ less than in controls. The fibres were more closely crowded together since in the thyrotoxic patients there were 398 fibres per sq. mm compared with 287 per sq. mm in controls (Ramsay, 1964).

Devic *et al.* (1947) described an alteration of the mitochondria in the region of the motor end plates. Coërs and Woolf (1959) using an intravital staining technique found changes in the terminal nerve fibres, mainly profuse distal sprouting, often with the formation of multiple end plates on single muscle fibres. Havard *et al.* (1963), using the same technique, found such abnormalities as diffuse axonal swellings with multiple beading, rounded or oval swellings of the terminal axon (Fig. 1.7) and clubbing of the end plate in 77% of their patients. Neither of the last two studies contained data pertaining to controls, so it is difficult to assess the significance of their findings.

Hed, Kirstein and Lundmark (1958) noticed the presence in the muscle tissue of iron-loaded phagocytes. The sub-sarcolemmal semi-lunar accumulations of acid-mucopolysaccharides observed by

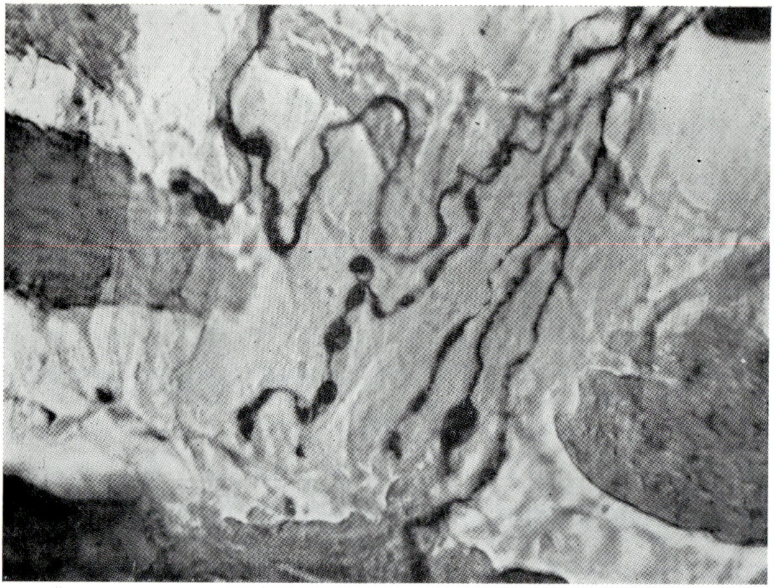

Figure 1.7(a). Biopsy from vastus medialis (×500: methylene blue) showing multiple axonal swellings of varying size and intensity of staining. (From Havard *et al.*, 1963).

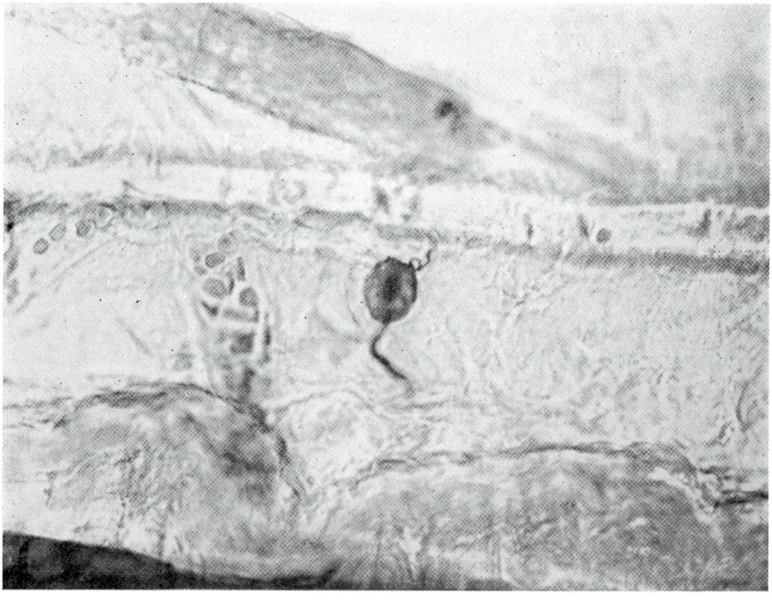

Figure 1.7(b). Biopsy from vastus medialis (×500: methylene blue) showing a large oval swelling of a terminal axon. (From Havard *et al.*, 1963).

Asböe-Hansen, Iversen and Wichmann (1953) in thyrotoxicosis, but most markedly in those with progressive exophthalmos, have been confirmed by Kirchheiner (1962), though Adams, Denny-Brown and Pearson (1962) were unable to find any. These histological features can only be seen in muscles which have been fixed in basic lead acetate; this precipitates acid-mucopolysaccharides (Iversen, Asböe-Hansen and Carlsen, 1953). Kirchheiner (1962) found these semi-lunar masses in 55% of thyrotoxics. Kroll and Kuwabara (1966), using the same method of fixation, were unable to find semi-lunar accumulations of mucopolysaccharides in the ocular muscles of exophthalmic patients.

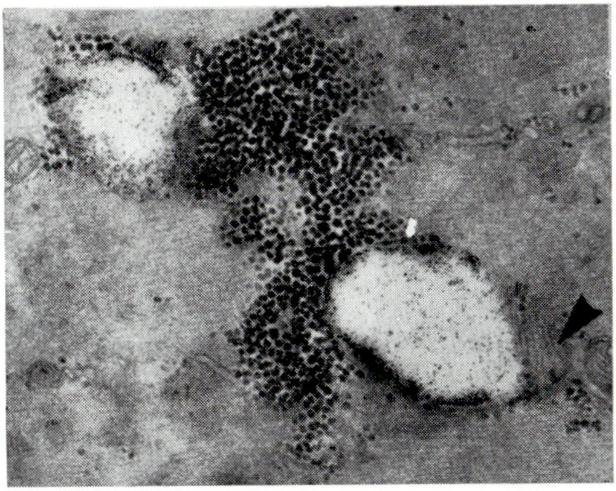

Figure 1.8. Electron micrograph (×20,000) of the quadriceps muscle of a 40-year-old woman with thyrotoxic myopathy. There is replacement of mitochondrial contents by amorphous and finely granular material. The arrow indicates a small remaining fragment of normal matrix and cristae in one mitochondrion. (From Engel, 1966).

Electron microscopy

Engel (1966) has described the electron microscopic appearance of the proximal muscles of two patients with thyrotoxicosis. On light microscopy the muscle fibres appeared normal, though there was a moderate increase in perimysial fatty connective tissue. On electron microscopy, however, many mitochondria showed structural alteration. There was partial replacement by light, amorphous material which contained scattered, small, dense granules (Fig. 1.8). In some mitochondria the granules were more dense and there were also membranous fragments and other debris (Fig. 1.9). Sometimes

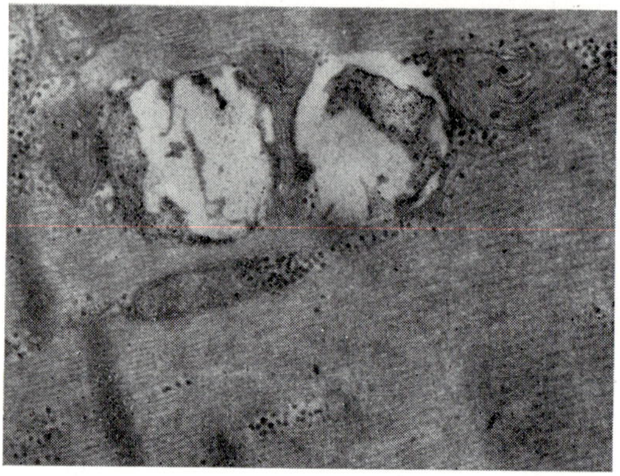

Figure 1.9. Electron micrograph (×20,000) of the deltoid muscle of a 45-year-old woman with thyrotoxic myopathy. The mitochondrion is filled with dense granular material, membranous fragments and debris. (From Engel, 1966).

structures which were almost certainly totally degenerate mitochondria were seen next to normal mitochondria (Fig. 1.10). In longitudinal sections some elongated mitochondria, up to 4 μ in length, were seen. Tsujihata (1969) in an electron microscopic study of 5 patients with thyrotoxic myopathy, found abnormal muscle mitochondria in all of them.

In Engel's (1966) study focal dilatation of the transverse tabular system were seen in some muscle fibres (Fig. 1.11), but the adjacent lateral vesicles and other components of the sarcoplasmic reticulum were normal. Both Tsujihata (1969) and Engel (1966) noted glycogen deposits in the muscle fibre. Engel thought that the subsarcolemmal deposits (Fig. 1.10) were the same as those described by Asböe-Hansen and his colleagues (1953) and by Kirchheiner (1962).

Experimental pathology

Rats treated with thyroxine become less active (Brody, 1941) and are less resistant to fatigue (Malcolm and Whitehead, 1944). Muscles exposed to excess thyroxine, in addition to being more fatigued, exert less force and use up relatively more oxygen (Schwartz and Lein, 1955; Schwartz *et al.*, 1960).

Gustafsson *et al.* (1965) studied the effects of anabolic doses of thyroid hormone on thyroidectomized rats. They found proliferation

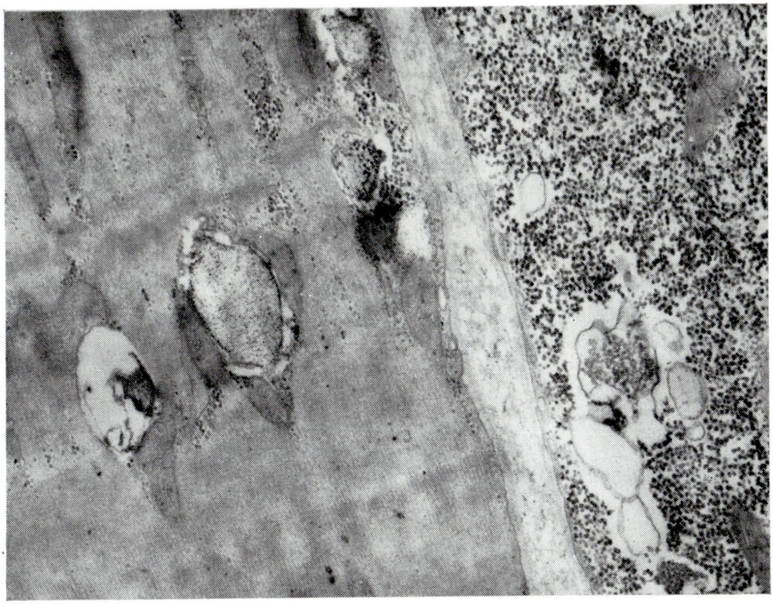

Figure 1.10. Electron micrograph (×20,700) of the same muscle as in Fig. 1.9. A vesicular body containing membranous fragments and debris and another containing dense granular and amorphous material are seen adjacent to normal mitochondrion. The fibre on the right contains a large subsarcolemmal glycogen deposit within which a few mitochondria and irregularly shaped vesicles are present. (From Engel, 1966).

of mitochondria and a quantity of mitochondria which was 2·5 to 3·5 times that of controls. It was frequently noted that the mitochondria abutted upon each other at points corresponding closely to the location of the transverse tubular system. The mitochondria showed closely packed cristae with an angular or zig-zag pattern and frequently small, dense granules were seen in the matrix. There is an interesting overlap between the work of Gustafsson and his co-workers and that of Engel, even though the former was done on anabolically hyperthyroid animals, while the latter was an examination of patients who were in a catabolic state. Both noted enlarged mitochondria and the presence of dense granular material in the mitochondria, though the changes were more marked in Engel's patients. O'Brien and Klitgaard (1965) found an increase in mitochondrial size, increased amounts of cristae and intramitochondrial

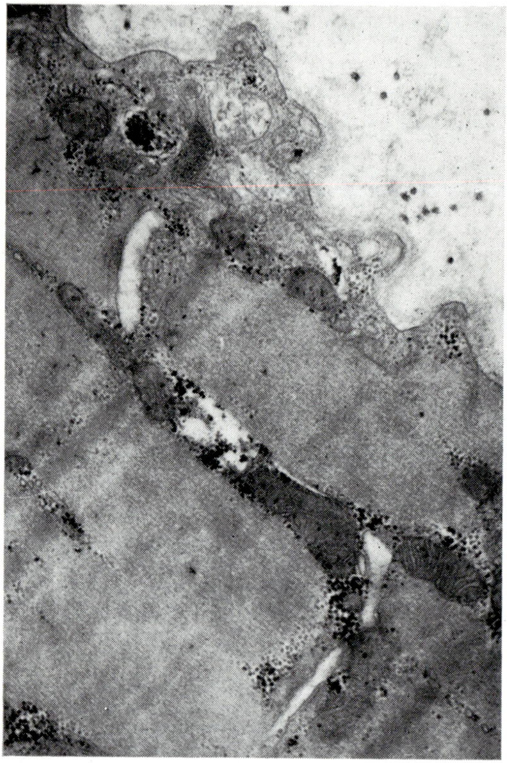

Figure 1.11. Electron micrograph of the same muscle as in Fig. 1.9. (×19,000). There is focal dilatation of the transverse tubular system. (From Engel, 1966).

deposits in rat livers from animals made hyperthyroid to a B.M.R. of 140% with L-thyroxine. Zaimis *et al.* (1968), working with cats and guinea pigs which had been given thyroxine found that the mitochondria of skeletal muscle were either enlarged or unfolded or showed both changes. The mitochondria showed a greater variation in their internal structure than normal and the main feature was more densely packed cristae. Thus, there is a remarkable similarity between the mitochondrial changes in the muscle and liver of different animals and in human muscle and it suggests that one of the prime effects of thyroxine is on mitochondrial structure.

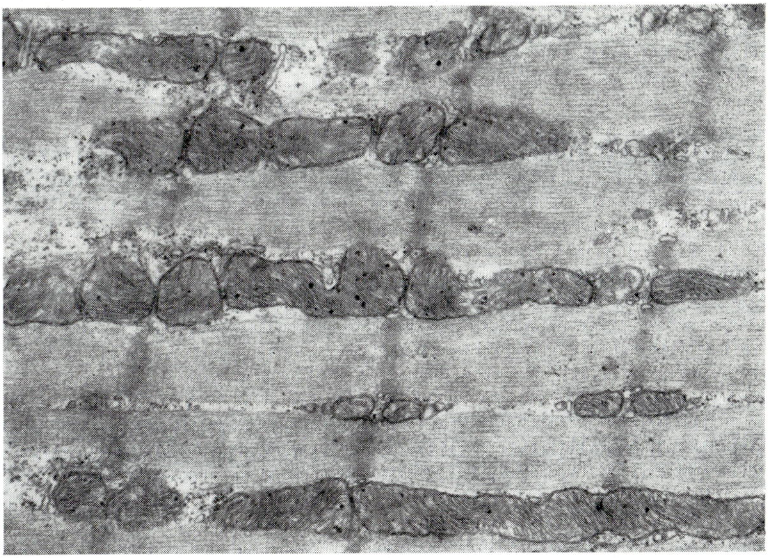

Figure 1.12. Electron micrograph of muscle fibre taken from a normal rat made hypermetabolic by treatment with L-thyroxine for three weeks. The interfibrillar mitochondria are elongated, one at the lower right of the the picture being over one sarcomere in length. The mitochondrial cristae are tightly packed and angulated and small dense granules are seen in the mitochondrial matrix. Magnification $\times$24,000.

(By courtesy of Dr. Björn Afzelius).

Relationship between structure and function

Mitochondria contain the oxidative enzymes of the citric acid cycle, which is the terminal oxidation chain, and of the phosphorylative mechanisms associated with them. The latter lead to the formation of adenosine-triphosphate (ATP) which is necessary for the process of muscle contraction. In muscles with persistent contractile activity such as maintaining posture against the force of gravity and in locomotion, energy metabolism is predominantly oxidative and the mitochondria are abundant. These are the muscles which in animals are composed predominantly of red or Type I fibres, have a slow response to stimulation and rely on oxidative phosphorylation as a primary source of energy. On the other hand, muscles which are used for rapid, intermittent voluntary movement, and which have a fast response to stimulation, are made up mainly of white or Type II fibres. These fibres contain very few mitochondria and little in the way of oxidative enzymes, but obtain most of their energy by glycolysis (for reviews see Sissons, 1969; Buller, 1969; Price, 1969).

In man it is probable that most muscles consist of a mixture of slow Type I fibres and fast Type II fibres. Dubowitz (1968) did not find any clearcut pattern of differences between proximal and distal muscles. Buchthal and Schmalbruch (1970) on the other hand showed that a muscle such as gastrocnemius, engaged frequently in sustained effort, contains 83% of Type I fibres, while a less strenuously used muscle, the triceps, has only 2% of Type I fibres. Man is similar to experimental animals in having a greater abundance of mitochondria in Type I than in Type II fibres (Engel and Macdonald, 1970). However, as the latter authors point out, information is lacking about the relative proportions of mitochondria in man for a given age, sex, muscle, fibre type and level of physical activity. Abnormal mitochondria have recently been implicated in the aetiology of several patients with myopathy, but without thyrotoxicosis (Luft *et al.*, 1962; Shy, Gonatas and Perez, 1966; Van Wijngaarden *et al.*, 1967; Spiro, Prineas and Moore, 1970; Haydar *et al.*, 1971). In two of the cases there was evidence of severe hypermetabolism.

Buchthal and Schmalbruch (1970) have shown an interesting correlation between the relative proportions of different fibre types and the contraction times of the muscles. In the long head of the biceps, with 25% Type I fibres, 30% of the contraction times measured were above 60 m sec. compared to only 2% in the triceps, a muscle which contained a mere 2% of Type I fibres. They found that during hypoxia, induced for between 30 and 45 minutes, contraction times became significantly shorter, compatible with the assumption that the slow Type I fibres, rich in mitochondria, consume more oxygen than the fast Type II fibres which depend more on anaerobic respiration for their energy supply. If there were a selective knockout of Type I fibres in thyrotoxicosis this would lead to a relative preponderance of fast Type II fibres. This might be at least partially responsible for the shortened Achilles tendon reflex. Peter and his colleagues (Peter, Worsfold and Stempel, 1970) have found increased amounts of sarcotubular vesicle in human thyrotoxic skeletal muscle. The sarcotubular vesicles of hyperthyroid rats showed an increased rate of calcium accumulation. It has already been noted that calcium concentrations are elevated in thyrotoxic muscle (p. 19). Since calcium plays an important role in the initiation of muscle contraction, this may also be an additional factor bringing about the rapidity of contraction of thyrotoxic muscle.

Aetiology of myopathy

Causative factors. Three possible factors must be considered in the aetiology of thyrotoxic myopathy. They are thyroid stimulating hormone (TSH), long-acting thyroid stimulator (LATS) and the thyroid hormones, thyroxine and triiodothyronine. Although the normal physiological role of TSH is to stimulate the thyroid gland, this does not happen in thyrotoxicosis; indeed, TSH is virtually absent from the blood of patients with this condition (Lemarchand-Béraud, Vanotti and Scazziga, 1967; Blum *et al.*, 1967) and can therefore be excluded as an aetiological agent. Long-acting thyroid stimulator has been demonstrated in up to 90% of patients with Graves' disease (Blum *et al.*, 1967) and it seems almost certain that this immunoglobulin, which behaves like a true antibody, is the agent which is responsible for the excessive production of thyroid hormone (Hetzel, 1968). However, since the myopathy always disappears after the successful treatment of hyperthyroidism, though significant amounts of circulating LATS may persist (Kriss, Pleshakov and Chien, 1964), it is difficult to incriminate this substance as a causative agent in muscle dysfunction. One comes to the inescapable conclusion that it is the excessive production of thyroid hormones which cause the muscle weakness. As has been noted earlier there is a close temporal relationship between the onset of the general symptoms of thyrotoxicosis and the symptoms of muscle weakness. The muscle wasting and the E.M.G. abnormalities all disappear when thyroid hormone levels are made normal (Havard *et al.*, 1963; Ramsay, 1965, 1966). Some of the mitochondrial changes were also seen to revert in experimental animals (Gustafsson *et al.*, 1965). Moreover there is ample experimental work showing that muscle weakness can be produced in animals by the administration of thyroxine and there have been instances of thyrotoxic myopathy induced in man by large doses of thyroid hormone.

It is possible that some of the histological changes found in thyrotoxic myopathy may not be due to excess thyroid hormone. Changes similar to those seen in thyrotoxic myopathy have been found in the extrinsic muscles of the eye in patients with thyrotoxicosis (Askanazy, 1898) and in patients with exophthalmos (Dudgeon and Urquhart, 1926). Dudgeon and Urquhart noticed a similarity between their findings and those of Buzzard (1905) in patients with myasthenia gravis. The same changes could be produced in the muscles of thyroidectomized guinea pigs by the injection of anterior pituitary extract (Paulson, 1939; Dobyns, 1946). Recently Pellegrini and

Scarlato (1970) have found both structural and biochemical changes in the skeletal muscles of euthyroid patients with ophthalmic Graves' disease. Histologically they found an increase in perimysial connective tissue, proliferation of sarcolemmal nuclei and occasional nuclei in the centre of muscle fibres. Acid phosphatase, not normally demonstrable in muscle, was found in all three cases as minute granules dispersed throughout the muscle fibres, with focal accumulations in the subsarcolemmal regions.

A substance, produced by the anterior pituitary, called "exophthalmos producing substance" (E.P.S.) may have something to do with the aetiology of exophthalmos (Kinderen, Houtstra-Lanz and Schwarz, 1960; Dobyns, Wright and Wilson, 1961; Kinderen, 1967). It may act synergistically with LATS (Kinderen, 1967), though some doubt its importance (Pimstone, Hoffenberg and Black, 1963). Kriss and his colleagues (1967) believe that the changes brought about in the extrinsic eye muscles in exophthalmos could be due to the deposition of a thyroid antigen–LATS complex.

It may therefore be wrong to ascribe all the histological changes seen in patients with thyrotoxic myopathy to the effects of excess thyroid hormone. Some may be due to either LATS, E.P.S. or both of them working synergistically. It would be interesting to discover whether patients with thyrotoxic myopathy due to a hyperfunctioning autonomous thyroid "hot" nodule have any histological changes apart from muscle fibre atrophy.

Why proximal myopathy?

While thyrotoxicosis causes muscle weakness in about 80% of patients, in less than 20% are the distal muscles involved (Havard *et al.*, 1963; Ramsay, 1965). Electromyographic changes indicative of a myopathy have been found in the proximal muscles in about 90% of the patients, but in only 43% of the patients did the distal muscles show any abnormalities (Ramsay, 1965). Every patient with an abnormal distal muscle E.M.G. had pronounced myopathic changes in the proximal muscle tested. Comparing these findings in unselected thyrotoxics with an analysis of the patients described in the literature as having "chronic thyrotoxic myopathy" one finds that all of the latter had proximal weakness, 34·3% had distal involvement and 16·4% had weakness of bulbar muscles (Ramsay, 1965). It should be noted that patients with bulbar muscle weakness always had involvement of both their proximal and distal skeletal muscles as well. The evidence points to there being a progressive susceptibility of the different groups of muscles to the thyrotoxic process, first proximal, then distal and finally bulbar. Extensor muscles in hyperthyroid patients were found to be twice as commonly affected as flexors (Ramsay, 1966).

The muscles most commonly involved in thyrotoxicosis are those mainly used for the maintenance of posture and during prolonged effort. Although the differences are not so clearcut as in lower animals, it is probable that these muscles contain relatively more red muscle fibres than white, while the opposite is true of the more rapidly contracting distal muscles which are used for intermittent movements (Adams, Denny-Brown and Pearson, 1962). Red muscle fibres contain far more mitochondria than do white (Lawrie, 1953) and the mitochondria are rich in such oxidative enzymes as lactic dehydrongenase, succinic dehydrogenase and cytochrome oxidase. White fibres contain few oxidative enzymes but relatively large amounts of phosphorylases which are concerned in anaerobic glycolysis (Sissons, 1969). The mitochondrial enzymes are involved in oxidative phosphorylation which results in the production of the high-energy phosphate bonds of adenosine-triphosphate (ATP) (Green, Loomis and Auerbach, 1948; Kennedy and Lehninger, 1949; Harman, 1950; Lehninger, 1959; Green and Hatefi, 1961). For every atom of oxygen utilized in the mitochondrion three ATP molecules are formed, giving a phosphate:oxygen (P:O) ratio of 3:1. This transformation of oxidative to phosphorylative bond energy has been called "coupling" by Loomis and Lipmann (1948). When the P:O ratio is 3:1, the system is said to be "tightly coupled".

Hoch (1962a, b) has shown that thyroid hormones have a biphasic action, being anabolic and energy-conserving in low doses, but catabolic and energy-wasting in large doses. He has summarized the evidence (1968) that in toxic amounts the thyroid hormones "uncouple" oxidative phosphorylative by a direct action on mitochondria' The result of this is a diminished production of ATP and a wastage of energy as heat. The thyrotoxic subject consumes more oxygen than normal and produces an excessive amount of heat, a fact which accounts for many of the signs and symptoms of thyrotoxicosis—vasodilatation, sweating, etc. In addition to the biochemical effects of the thyroid hormones in the experimental situation, physiological amounts of thyroxine have been shown to cause swelling of mitochondria *in vivo* and *in vitro*, an increase in the absolute amount of mitochondria and an increase in the cristae mitochondriales (Tapley, 1964).

Alterations in mitochondrial structure were first noticed by Devic *et al.*, in 1947 in muscle taken from thyrotoxic patients and more recently Engel (1966) has found degenerating mitochondria in electron microscope preparations. The swollen mitochondria were found to contain decreased amounts of ATP (Tapley, 1964). Chappell and Greville (1958) have shown that the thyroxine-induced swelling of mitochondria can be reversed by the addition of ATP to the *in vitro* preparation. Satoyoshi and his colleagues (1963a) found a decreased amount of ATP in muscle taken from thyrotoxic patients and were able to show a relationship between those diminished levels and the loss of muscular strength of their patients. Other authors have put forward alternative theories as to the reasons for the inefficient utilization of energy in thyrotoxicosis. Peter and his colleagues (1970) demonstrated an increase in the yield of mitochondria from the muscles of thyrotoxic patients and thought that this partly accounted for the hypermetabolism. Smith (1964) postulated that thyroxine may stimulate pathways whereby reduced diphosphopyridine nucleotide and triphosphopyridine nucleotides are oxidized outside the mitochondria by poorly phosphorylating transfers or within the mitochondria at lower levels in the respiratory chain. The result is the production of only one molecule of ATP instead of three; the remainder is lost as heat. Stocker, Samaha and De Groot (1968) thought that the defect could lie either in the utilization of ATP or merely in an acceleration of the normal processes of oxidative phosphorylation.

Apart from oxidative phosphorylation there is another source of muscle ATP—the phosphoryl group donated by phosphocreatine. This, however, is only sufficient for a very short time—just a few contractions—and must itself be resynthesized from creatine via mitochondrial mechanisms. Phosphocreatine kinase is inhibited by excess thyroxine (Askonas, 1951) and cellular potassium depletion which has been found in hyperthyroidism also adversely affects the manufacture of phosphocreatine (Grob, Liljestrand and Johns, 1957; Satoyoshi *et al.*, 1963a). Both factors contribute to a diminished availability of ATP. Satoyoshi *et al.* (1963a) found a reduction of phosphocreatine in thyrotoxic muscle. The inability of the cells to resynthesize phosphocreatine is reflected in the raised serum levels (Kuhlbäck, 1957; Satoyoshi *et al.*, 1963a), and the increased urinary excretion of creatine. The reduced tolerance of thyrotoxic patients to ingested creatine has even been made the basis of a test for the disease (Thorn and Eder, 1946; Wilkins and Fleischmann, 1946).

Thyrotoxic muscles show a diminished uptake of creatine (Kuhlbäck, 1957). Creatine normally undergoes anhydration to creatine in the muscles. In thyrotoxicosis there is a decreased production of creatinine and this is reflected in lowered serum and urine levels (Kuhlbäck, 1957).

The occasional finding of a low or absent excretion of creatine in some patients (Zierler, 1951) was attributed by Hoch (1962a) to a failure of heptatic synthesis of creatine. This requires the ATP dependent transfer of a methyl group from methionine to glycocyamine.

Muscle normally contracts as a result of the calcium-induced dephosphorylation of ATP which causes activity at the cross linkages between actin and myosin (Mommaerts, 1963; Price, 1969). Probably because there is a shortage of ATP in thyrotoxicosis, the force of contraction becomes diminished (Plummer and Boothby, 1923; Smith and Whalen, 1960).

This lack of ATP probably also explains why the energy-dependent control of membrane permeability breaks down. Green and Matty (1962) showed a thyroxine-induced increase in permeability to water, and an increase in muscle cell water in patients with thyrotoxic myopathy was found by Staffurth and Thompson (1965). The loss of selective permeability may also account for the finding of a 21% reduction in potassium and a two-fold increase in muscle fibre sodium, as well as a decrease in aldolase and lactic dehydrogenase (Satoyoshi *et al.*, 1963a).

Although it seems likely that the prime effect of thyroid hormones on muscle is mediated via their action on the mitochondria, structural changes in the muscle fibre may also play a part. For example, Engel (1966), using an electron microscope, has found alterations in the muscle cell surface and of the transverse tubular system which is important in the local activation of the striated muscle fibre (Huxley and Taylor, 1958).

The fact that it takes about two months for the patients to recover normal muscle strength after the start of effective antithyroid treatment (Ramsay, 1966) argues in favour of there being a structural alteration in the muscle fibre in addition to a biochemical derangement. The enlarged mitochondria of thyrotoxicosis persist for some months in experimental animals (Gustafsson *et al.*, 1965).

The role of catecholamines in thyrotoxic myopathy

It is well known that many of the peripheral manifestations of thyrotoxicosis are similar to those produced by catecholamines (Gifford *et al.*, 1964) and it is thought that in some way excess thyroid hormone potentiates the effects of normal circulating amounts of catecholamines. This may be mediated via the enzyme adenyl cyclase, the synthesis of which is increased by thyroid hormone (Brodie *et al.*, 1966). Adenyl cyclase is activated by catecholamines; indeed Sutherland and his colleagues (Robison, Butcher and Sutherland, 1967) have suggested that adenyl cyclase may be the β adrenergic receptor. Marsden and Meadows (1970) have shown that adrenaline shortens the duration of the slow calf muscle twitch. That this is due to stimulation of β adrenergic receptors was proved by the abolition of the effect by the intra-arterial administration of the β adrenergic antagonist D–L propranolol. This might fit in with the finding by Pimstone, Marine and Pimstone (1968) of improvement in the muscle strength of 5 out of 8 patients with thyrotoxic myopathy with the administration of propranolol. They argued that the effect of excessive adenyl cyclase activity would lead to an increase in cyclic adenosine monophosphate (cyclic AMP) synthesis from ATP. The cyclic AMP would then stimulate ATP dependent metabolic pathways via enzymes such as phosphorylase and lipase. The net result would be that, in a situation where the supply of ATP was already diminished by a decrease in oxidative phosphorylation, stimulation of adenyl cyclase production would cause a further fall in ATP. This situation would therefore be expected to be improved to some extent by propranolol which blocks the effects of adrenergic stimulation.

Differential diagnosis of thyrotoxic myopathy

In many cases of thyrotoxicosis in which muscle wasting and weakness are the presenting features, the diagnosis will be easy to make because of the presence of the other well-known features of Graves' disease, particularly the exophthalmos and the enlarged thyroid gland. The difficulty usually arises in elderly patients with "masked" thyrotoxicosis. They may be diagnosed as having carcinomatous myopathy, cachexia or polymyositis and unless the possible significance of atrial fibrillation is appreciated and the appropriate thyroid function tests are done, the diagnosis may be long delayed. Contrary to some current belief (Ingbar and Woeber, 1968) thyrotoxic myopathy does occur in patients with solitary autonomous hyperfunctioning thyroid adenomas (Logothetis and Warner, 1962; Ramsay *et al.*, 1972). Careful palpation of the neck will usually reveal the nodule.

Prognosis. Two of the earlier patients in the literature described as having "thyrotoxic myopathy" died of respiratory paralysis (Morgan and Williams, 1940; McEachern and Ross, 1942) which might have been due to involvement of the respiratory muscles (Massey *et al.*, 1967), though it is possible that they could have had myasthenia gravis (Millikan and Haines, 1953). A patient of Thorn and Eder (1946), with some evidence of bulbar involvement, succumbed. Three patients of Devic *et al.* (1947) died following thyroidectomy, but apart from one person (Hed, Kirstein and Lundmark, 1958), who died of an unrelated disease, death in a patient with chronic thyrotoxic myopathy has not been reported since 1947. This reflects the introduction of safer and more effective treatment for hyperthyroidism in the last 25 years.

Full recovery of muscle strength was noted in 53 of 76 patients reported in the literature, and full power returned in 100% of thyrotoxic patients in recent series (Havard *et al.*, 1963; Satoyoshi *et al.*, 1963a, b; Ramsay, 1964, 1966). Muscle power became normal in about the same time (mean 2·2 months) as it took for the patients to become euthyroid (mean 2·1 months) after the start of treatment, although atrophy took slightly longer (mean 2·8 months) to disappear (Ramsay, 1966). Even in patients described with proximal, distal and bulbar muscle involvement there was complete recovery of muscular strength after successful treatment of thyrotoxicosis (Joasoo *et al.*, 1970). Creatine and creatinine excretion returned to normal (Ramsay, 1966) as did electromyograms (Havard *et al.*, 1963; Coomes, 1965; Ramsay, 1965; Yates, 1965).

Treatment. Since virtually all patients with thyrotoxicosis have a myopathy it is wise to hold off the question of thyroid surgery for at least three months after the initiation of adequate antithyroid therapy. Deaths due to respiratory failure have been described and there are occasional cases where patients prepared for thyroid surgery only with iodine have had difficulty in re-establishing spontaneous respiration post-operatively (Ramsay, 1970). This suggests that in some patients the respiratory muscles are myopathic (Massey *et al.*, 1967).

No matter what form of treatment is used to render the patient euthyroid the muscle weakness will disappear shortly after the achievement of the euthyroid state. Pimstone and his colleagues (1968) claimed that treatment with propranolol improved the muscle weakness in just over half of their small series, but their results have not yet been confirmed.

ACUTE THYROTOXIC MYOPATHY

A number of reports have appeared of muscle weakness of seemingly acute onset in patients with thyrotoxicosis (Laurent, 1944; Waldenström, 1945, Sheldon and Walker, 1946; Strong, 1949; Gimlette, 1959; Logothetis and Warner, 1962). Waldenström (1945), in addition to his own cases, drew attention to a large number of similar ones described in the German literature of the previous 50 years. The history was nearly always one of the sudden onset of a bulbar palsy in a patient who had had previous symptoms of thyrotoxicosis for several months or even years. It is apparent that in most of the cases the thyrotoxicosis was extremely severe. Many of Waldenström's (1945) cases had diarrhoea and vomiting and thyrotoxic crisis or coma, which has also been noticed in subsequent reports (Chapman and Maloof, 1956; Gimlette, 1959; Heinrich *et al.*, 1962). Eighty per cent of Waldenström's personal cases had atrial fibrillation compared with only 14% in a series of unselected thyrotoxic patients (Ramsay, 1964), indicating the severity of the thyrotoxicosis. In addition to ptosis, difficulty with speech, dysphagia and nasal regurgitation of fluids, it is clear from the reports published since 1945 that there was also generalized muscle weakness; exophthalmic ophthalmoplegia was not a common feature, occurring in only two cases (Waldenström, 1945; Strong, 1949) out of 55 (3·6%). Strong (1949) found only oedema in biopsies of extraocular and temporal muscles, though Gimlette (1959) described widespread degeneration of muscle fibres and the presence of lymphorrhages. Electromyography has been done on only 3 of these patients and in all of the cases the picture was that of a myopathy. Most of the earlier patients succumbed, but Waldenström (1945) was able to get a full remission in his patients using iodine followed by partial thyroidectomy. Subsequently, complete recovery has been obtained in all cases with medical therapy, using antithyroid drugs or radioactive iodine (Strong, 1949; Chapman and Maloof, 1956; Gimlette, 1959; Heinrich *et al.*, 1962; Logothetis and Warner, 1962).

There seems little doubt that severely thyrotoxic patients may also show such diffuse abnormalities in the central nervous system as paraphasia, acalculia and psychosis with hallucinations (Waldenström, 1945; Greer and Parsons, 1968). Degeneration and hæmorrhage into the cranial nerve nuclei was found in 3 early cases (Waldenström, 1945) and slight to moderate swelling of oligodendroglia in the sub-cortical white matter was described by Chapman and Maloof (1956) in one patient. Heinrich and his colleagues (1962) found clinical evidence of an upper motor neurone lesion in their patient. Probably this small group of patients with cerebral and brain stem symptoms and signs should be called "thyrotoxic encephalopathy". Obviously one must consider whether the bulbar palsies could be of nuclear origin. However, it has been already noted that these patients had evidence of preceding skeletal muscle weakness and it has been remarked upon earlier that, of all the patients described in the literature as having "chronic thyrotoxic myopathy", 16·4% also had bulbar muscle involvement. Moreover, Joasoo, Murray and Steinbeck (1970) have recently described 12 patients with thyrotoxic bulbar muscle weakness, all of whom had evidence of proximal myopathy.

Since full recovery takes place when prompt treatment is initiated, it would seem unlikely that there could have been any significant damage to cranial nerve nuclei and it seems more likely that these patients, too, suffered a reversible derangement of bulbar muscle function in addition to their skeletal muscle disease. "Acute thyrotoxic myopathy" may represent the stage at which bulbar muscle weakness complicates "chronic thyrotoxic myopathy". If the disease is severe enough it would not be surprising if the stage of generalized weakness was short and the bulbar involvement, with its dramatic and life threatening symptoms, became the most pronounced feature. This is illustrated by the case reported by Logothetis and Warner (1962). The patient, a woman aged 63, had had weakness of her legs for two years. Her condition became suddenly worse over a period of seven days. In addition to a proximal myopathy affecting arms and legs she was found to have ptosis, facial weakness, nearly complete loss of extraocular movements and poor movement of the palate and tongue. The cause of her thyrotoxicosis was a thyroid adenoma. Although her serum potassium was reduced at 2·5 m Eq/l, intravenous potassium therapy made no difference to her weakness; nor did the administration of edrophonium (Tensilon). A muscle biopsy of the deltoid showed muscle fibre atrophy and adipose tissue replacement. Electromyography performed on several muscles showed evidence of a myopathy. There was nothing on EMG to suggest myasthenia gravis and there were no signs of denervation. She was treated initially by radioactive iodine followed after a few days by potassium iodide and methimazole. Within five weeks her ophthalmoplegia and bulbar weakness had disappeared, though she still had skeletal muscle weakness. Three weeks later this too was judged to have returned to normal. Six months later the woman died of a cerebellar haemorrhage and microscopy of the brain stem was found to be normal.

It must be remembered, however, that there is a possibility of myasthenia gravis in this group of patients. Millikan and Haines (1953) thought that many of the cases in the early literature were probably examples of coincident myasthenia gravis and thyrotoxicosis. Neostigmine certainly gave dramatic relief in three more recent cases of acute thyrotoxic bulbar palsy (Laurent, 1944; Sheldon and Walker, 1946) and it is therefore mandatory to try the effect of edrophonium or neostigmine on any thyrotoxic patient who presents with a bulbar palsy, particularly if there is ptosis.

REFERENCES

Abraham, A. S., Atkinson, M. and Roscoe, B. (1966). Value of ankle jerk timing in the assessment of thyroid function. *Brit. med. J.*, *i*, 830.

Adams, R. D., Denny-Brown, D. and Pearson, C. M. (1962). "Diseases of Muscle". A Study in Pathology. Kimpton, London.

Adrian, E. D. and Gelfan, S. (1933). Rhythmic activity in skeletal muscle fibres. *J. Physiol.* (*Lond.*), **78,** 271.

Araki, S., Terao, A., Matsumoto, I., Narazaki, T. and Kuroiwa, Y. (1968). Muscle cramps in chronic thyrotoxic myopathy. Report of a case. *Arch. Neurol.* (*Chic.*), **19,** 315.

Asböe-Hansen, G., Iversen, K. and Wichmann, R. (1952). Malignant exophthalmos; muscular changes and thyrotropin content in serum. *Acta endocr.* (*Kbh.*), **11,** 376.

Asböe-Hansen, G., Iversen, K. and Wichmann, R. (1953). Progressive exophthalmos; muscular changes and thyrotropin content of serum. *Ugeskr. Laeg.*, **115,** 889.

Askanazy, M. (1898). Pathologisch-anatomische Beiträge zur Kenntniss des Morbus Basedowii, insbesondere über die dabei auftretende Muskelkrankung. *Dtsch. Arch. klin. Med.*, **61,** 118.

Askonas, B. A. (1951). Effect of thyroxine on creatine phosphokinase activity. *Nature* (*Lond.*), **167,** 933.

Asper, S. P. Jnr. and Wilson, E. H. (1957). Hyperthyroidism and infertility. *Brit. med. J.*, *i*, 1300.

Ayer, J. B., Means, J. H. and Lerman, J. (1934). Simulation of progressive muscular atrophy by exophthalmic goiter. *Endocrinology*, **18,** 701.

Bartels, E. C. and Pizer, E. (1944). Muscular atrophy in hyperthyroidism; report of a case. *Lahey Clin. Bull.*, **4,** 52.

Basedow, C. A. von (1840). Exophthalmos durch Hypertrophie des Zellgewebes in der Augenhöhle. *Wschr. ges. Heilk.*, **6,** 197.

Bathurst, L. W. (1895). A case of Graves' disease associated with idiopathic muscular atrophy; remarks. *Lancet*, *ii*, 529.

Blum, A. S., Greenspan, F. S., Hardgadine, J. R. and Lowenstein, J. M. (1967). Simultaneous detection of thyroid stimulating hormone (TSH) and long-acting thyroid stimulator (LATS). *Metabolism*, **16,** 960.

Boström, H. and Hed, R. (1958). Thyrotoxic myopathy and polymyositis in elderly patients; differential diagnostic viewpoints. *Acta med. scand.*, **162,** 225.

Brodie, B. B., Davies, J. I., Hynie, S., Krishna, G. and Weiss, B. (1966). Interrelationships of catecholamines with other endocrine systems. *Pharmacol. Rev.*, **18,** 273.

Brody, E. B. (1941). Influence of thyroidectomy on variability of neuromuscular activity in the rat. *Endocrinology*, **29,** 916.

Brody, T. M., Hurwitz, R. and Bain, J. A. (1954). Magnesium and effect of tetracycline antibiotics on oxidative process in mitochondria. *Antibiot. Chemother.*, **4,** 864.

Buchthal, F. (1957). In "An Introduction to Electromyography". Glydendal, Copenhagen.

Buchthal, F. (1970). Electrophysiological abnormalities in metabolic myopathies and neuropathies. In "Proceedings of the Nineteenth Congress of Scandinavian Neurologists", edited by P. Juul-Jensen, *Acta Neurologica Scandinavia*, **46,** Suppl. 43, p. 129.

Buchthal, F. and Pinelli, P. (1953). Muscle action potentials in polymyositis. *Neurology* (*Minneapolis*), **3,** 424.

Buchthal, F. and Rosenfalck, P. (1955). Action potential parameters in different human muscles. *Acta psychiat. neurol. Scand.*, **30,** 125.

Buchthal, F. and Rosenfalck, P. (1963). In "Muscular Dystrophy in Man and Animals". Edited by G. H. Bourne and M. N. Golarz, p. 193. Karger, Basel.

Buchthal, F. and Schmalbruch, H. (1970). Contraction times and fibre types in normal and diseased human muscle. In "Proceedings of an International Congress on Muscle Diseases, Milan, 1969". Edited by J. N. Walton, N. Canal and G. Scarlato, p. 131, Excerpta Medica, Amsterdam.

Buller, A. J. (1969). In "Disorders of Voluntary Muscle". Edited by J. N. Walton, p. 17. Churchill, London.

Buzzard, E. F. (1905). The clinical history and post-mortem examination of five cases of myasthenia gravis. *Brain*, **28,** 438.

Cachera, R., Lamotte, M., Darnis, F. and Raynaud, J. (1949a). Le volume des liquides extra-cellulaires dans l'hyperthyroïdie. *Sem. Hôp. Paris*, **25,** 1659.

Cachera, R., Lamotte, M., Darnis, F. and Raynaud, J. (1949b). Action du traitment de l'hyperthyroïdie sur les liquides extra-cellulaires. *Sem. Hôp. Paris*, **25,** 1666.

Chaney, W. C. (1924). Tendon reflexes in myxedema: a valuable aid in diagnosis. *J. Amer. med. Ass.*, **82,** 2013.

Chapman, E. M. and Maloof, F. (1956). Bizarre clinical manifestations of hyperthyroidism. *New Engl. J. Med.*, **254,** 1.

Chappell, J. B. and Greville, G. D. (1958). Mitochondrial swelling and its reversal. *Proc. 4th int. Congr. Biochem., Vienna*, **15,** 71.

Coërs, C. and Woolf, A. L. (1959). In "The Innervation of Muscle: A Biopsy Study", p. 118. Blackwell Scientific Publications, Oxford.

Collings, H. and Lienhard, W. F. (1957). Thyrotoxic myopathy with disturbance of potassium metabolism. *Neurology* (*Minneap.*), **7,** 667.

Coomes, E. N. (1965). The rate of recovery of reversible myopathies and the effects of anabolic agents in steroid myopathy. *Neurology* (*Minneap.*), **15,** 523.

Crooks, J., Murray, I. P. C. and Wayne, E. J. (1959). Statistical methods applied to the clinical diagnosis of thyrotoxicosis. *Quart. J. Med.*, **28,** 211.

Del Castillo, E. B., de la Balze, F. A. and Caul, H. (1940). Atrofia muscular e hipertiroidismo. *Semana med.*, **1,** 1110.

Del Castillo, J. and Katz, B. (1954a). The effect of magnesium on the activity of motor nerve endings. *J. Physiol.*, **124,** 553.

Del Castillo, J. and Katz, B. (1954b). Changes in end plate activity produced by pre-synaptic polarisation. *J. Physiol.*, **124,** 586.

Devic, A., Froment, R., Guinet, P. and Devic, M. (1947). Les dystrophies musculaires hyperthyroïdiennes. À propos de 14 observations personnelles de myopathie basedowienne. *J. Méd. Lyon*, **28,** 155.

Devic, A., Froment, R., Jeune, M. and Duverne, J. (1942). De l'existence d'une Myopathie Basedowienne. *Rev. neurol.* (*Paris*), **74,** 96.

Dobyns, B. W. (1945). Influence of thyroidectomy on the prominence of the eyes in guinea pig and in man. *Surg. Gynec. Obstet.*, **80,** 526.

Dobyns, B. W. (1946). Studies on exophthalmos produced by thyrotropic hormone. *Surg. Gynec. Obstet.*, **82,** 290.

Dobyns, B. M., Wright, A. and Wilson, L. (1961). Assay of the exophthalmos-producing substance in the serum of patients with progressive exophthalmos. *J. clin. Endocr.*, **21,** 648.

Dubowitz, V. (1968). Further studies on fibre types in skeletal muscle. In "Research in Muscular Dystrophy". Edited by Members of the Research Committee of the Muscular Dystrophy Group, p. 100. Pitman, London.

Dudgeon, L. S. and Urquhart, A. L. (1926). Lymphorrhages in the muscles in exophthalmic goitre. *Brain*, **49,** 182.

Eaton, L. M. and Lambert, E. H. (1957). Electromyography and electric stimulation of nerves in diseases of the motor unit; observations on myasthenic syndrome associated with malignant tumors. *J. Amer. med. Ass.*, **163,** 1117.

Ekbom, K., Hed, R., Herdenstam, C-G. P. and Nygren, A. (1966). The serum creatine phosphokinase activity and the Achilles reflex in hyperthyroidism and hypothyroidism. *Acta med. scand.*, **179,** 433.

Ellis, D. S. and Carey, W. (1961). Severe thyrotoxicosis with myopathy. *Amer. Practit.*, **12,** 517.

Engel, A. G. (1966). Electron microscopic observations in thyrotoxic and corticosteroid induced myopathies. *Mayo Clin. Proc.*, **41,** 785.

Engel, A. G. and MacDonald, R. D. (1970). Ultrastructural reactions in muscle disease and their light-microscopic correlates. In "Proceedings of an International Congress on Muscle Diseases". Milan, 1969. Edited by J. N. Walton, N. Canal and G. Scarlato, p. 71. Excerpta Medica, Amsterdam.

Engstrom, W. W. and Mason, H. L. (1944). The excretion of 17 ketosteroids in patients with hyperthyroidism and myxedema. *J. clin. Endocr.*, **4,** 517.

Froment, R., Gallavardin, L. and Devic, A. (1946). Myopathie révélatrice d'une maladie de Basedow et curable par l'aminothiazol. *J. Méd. Lyon*, **27,** 741.

Gifford, R. W., Kvale, W. F., Maher, F. T., Roth, G. M. and Priestley, J. T. (1964). Clinical features, diagnosis and treatment of pheochromocytoma: a review of 76 cases. *Mayo Clin. Proc.*, **39,** 281.

Gilson, W. E. (1959). Achilles reflex recording with a simple photomotograph. *New Engl. J. Med.*, **260,** 1027.

Gimlette, T. M. D. (1959). The muscular lesion in hyperthyroidism. *Brit. med. J.*, *ii*, 1143.

Graig, F. A. and Smith, J. C. (1965). Serum creatinine phosphokinase activity in altered thyroid states. *J. clin. Endocr. Metab.*, **25,** 723.

Graves, R. J. (1835). Clinical lectures. *Lond. med. surg. J.*, **7,** 516.

Green, D. E. and Hatefi, Y. (1961). The mitochondrion and biochemical machines. *Science*, **133,** 13.

Green, D. E., Loomis, W. F. and Auerbach, V. H. (1948). Studies on the cyclophorase system. I. The complete oxidation of pyruvic acid to carbon dioxide and water. *J. biol. Chem.*, **172,** 389.

Green, K. and Matty, A. J. (1962). Effect of thyroxine on the permeability of the isolated toad bladder. *Nature* (*Lond.*), **194,** 1190.

Greer, S. and Parsons, V. (1968). Schizophrenia-like psychosis in thyroid crisis. *Brit. J. Psychiat.*, **114,** 1357.

Griffiths, P. D. (1965). Serum enzymes in diseases of the thyroid gland. *J. clin. Path.*, **18,** 660.

Grob, D., Liljestrand, A. and Johns, R. J. (1957). Potassium movement in normal subjects. Effect on muscle function. *Amer. J. Med.*, **23,** 340.

Gustafsson, R., Tata, J. R., Lindberg, O. and Ernster, L. (1965). The relationship between the structure and activity of rat skeletal muscle mitochondria after thyroidectomy and thyroid hormone treatment *J. Cell Biol.*, **26,** 555.

Hamfelt, A. and Wetterberg, L. (1964). Thyrotoxic myopathy and Vitamin B6 metabolism. Report of a case with hyperthyroidism and periodic paralysis. *Acta neurol. scand.*, **40,** 386.

Harman, J. B. and Richardson, A. T. (1954). Generalised myokymia in thyrotoxicosis. Report of a case. *Lancet*, *ii*, 473.

Harman, J. W. (1950). Studies on mitochondria: I. The association of cyclophorase with mitochondria. *Exp. Cell Res.*, **1,** 382.

Havard, C. W. H. (1962). Thyrotoxic myopathy; a reappraisal and report of three cases. *Brit. med. J.*, *i*, 440.

Havard, C. W. H., Campbell, E. D. R., Ross, H. B. and Spence, A. W. (1963). Electromyographic and histological findings in the muscles of patients with thyrotoxicosis. *Quart. J. Med.*, **32,** 145.

Haydar, N. A., Conn, H. L., Afifi, A., Wakid, N., Ballas, S. and Fawaz, K. (1971). Severe hypermetabolism with primary abnormality of skeletal muscle mitochondria. *Ann. intern. med.*, **74,** 548.

Hed, R., Kirstein, L. and Lundmark, C. (1958). Thyrotoxic myopathy. *J. Neurol. Neurosurg. Psychiat.*, **21,** 270.

Heinrich, W. D., McCabe, E. B., Nicely, D. A. and Elder, J. C. (1962). Encephalopathic hyperthyroidism manifesting as as dysphagia. *Amer. J. Roentgenol.*, **88,** 336.

Hess, J. W., MacDonald, R. P., Frederick, R. J., Jones, R. N., Neely, J. and Gross, D. (1964). Serum creatine phosphokinase (CPK) activity in disorders of heart and skeletal muscle. *Ann. intern. Med.*, **61,** 1015.

Hetzel, B. S. (1968). The aetiology and pathogenesis of hyperthyroidism. *Postgrad. med. J.*, **44,** 363.

Hoch, F. L. (1962a). Thyrotoxicosis as a disease of mitochondria. *New Engl. J. Med.*, **266,** 446 and 498.

Hoch, F. L. (1962b). Biochemical actions of thyroid hormones. *Physiol. Rev.*, **42,** 605.

Hoch, F. L. (1968). Biochemistry of hyperthyroidism and hypothyroidism. *Postgrad. med. J.*, **44,** 347.

Hoffenburg, R. and Eales, L. (1956). Chronic thyrotoxic myopathy; a report of two cases. *S. Afr. med. J.*, **30,** 1246.

Huxley, A. F. and Taylor, R. E. (1958). Local activation of striated muscle fibres. *J. Physiol.* (*Lond.*), **144,** 426.

Ingbar, S. H. and Woeber, K. A. (1968). In "Textbook of Endocrinology", edited by R. H. Williams, p. 228. Saunders, Philadelphia.

Iversen, K., Asböe-Hansen, G. and Carlsen, F. (1953). Electron microscopy of certain muscle lesions in patients with pituitary-thyroid disorders. *Acta Endocr.* (*Kbh.*), **14,** 177.

Jenkinson, D. H. (1957). The nature of the antagonism between calcium and magnesium ions at the neuromuscular junction. *J. Physiol.*, **138,** 434.

Joasoo, A., Murray, I. P. C. and Steinbeck, A. W. (1970). Involvement of bulbar muscles in thyrotoxic myopathy. *Aust. Ann. Med.*, **19,** 338.

Jungers, P. and Savoie, J.-C. (1963). Étude du potassium échangeable dans l'hyperthyroïdie, à l'aide du ^{42}K. *Revue Française d'Études Cliniques et Bibliogiques*, **8,** 773.

Kennedy, E. P. and Lehninger, A. L. (1949). Oxidation of fatty acids and tricarboxylic acid cycle intermediates by isolated rat liver mitochondria. *J. biol. Chem.*, **179,** 957.

Kinderen, P. J. Der (1967). EPS, LATS and exophthalmos. In "Thyrotoxicosis". Proceedings of an International Symposium, Edinburgh, edited by W. J. Irvine, p. 221. Livingstone, Edinburgh.

Kinderen, P. J. Der, Houtstra-Lanz, M. and Schwarz, F. (1960). Exophthalmos-producing substance in human serum. *J. clin. Endocr.*, **20,** 712.

Kirchheiner, B. (1962). Specific muscle lesions in pituitary-thyroid disorders. *Acta med. scand.*, **172,** 539.

Kite, W. C., McClintock, J. C. and Graves, R. W. (1954). Chronic thyrotoxic myopathy. *N.Y. St. J. Med.*, **54,** 1613.

Kleeman, C. R., Epstein, F. H., McKay, D. and Taborsky, E. (1958). Effects of hypo- and hyperthyroidism on the filterability of serum magnesium. *J. clin. Endocrinol. Metab.*, **18,** 1111.

Kobayashi, A. and Takeuchi, K. (1967). Magnesium levels and thyroid disease. *Lancet*, *ii*, 1152.

Kriss, J. P., Pleshakov, V. and Chien, J. R. (1964). Isolation and identification of the long acting thyroid stimulator and its relation to hyperthyroidism and circumscribed pre-tibial myxedema. *J. clin. Endocr.*, **24,** 1005.

Kroll, A. J. and Kuwabara, T. (1966). Dysthyroid ocular myopathy. Anatomy, histology and electron microscopy. *Arch. Ophthal.* (*Chicago*), **76,** 244.

Kuhlbäck, B. (1957). Creatine and creatinine metabolism in thyrotoxicosis and hypothyroidism. A clinical study. *Acta med. scand.*, **159,** Supp. 331.

Lahey, F. H. (1931). Apathetic thyroidism. *Ann. Surg.*, **93,** 1026.

Lahey, F. H. (1926). Quadriceps test for the myasthenia of thyroidism. *J. Amer. med. Ass.*, **87,** 754.

Lambert, E. H., Underdahl, L. O., Beckett, S. and Mederos, L. O. (1951). A study of the ankle jerk in myxedema. *J. clin. Endocrinol.*, **11,** 1186.

Laurent, L. P. E. (1944). Acute thyrotoxic bulbar palsy. *Lancet*, *i*, 87.

Lawrie, R. A. (1953). The relation of energy-rich phosphate in muscle to myoglobin and to cytochrome-oxidase activity. *Biochem. J.*, **55,** 305.

Lawson, J. D. (1958). The free Achilles reflex in hypothyroidism and hyperthyroidism. *New Engl. J. Med.*, **259,** 761.

Lawson, J. D. and Weissbein, A. S. (1959). The free Achilles reflex during treatment of hyperthyroidism. *Amer. J. med. Sci.*, **238,** 39.

Leeper, R. D. (1963). Effect of thyroid hormone on human serum ribonuclease. *J. clin. Endocr.*, **23,** 426.

Lehninger, A. L. (1959). Respiratory energy transformation. In "Biophysical Sciences: A Study Programme". Edited by J. L. Oncley, F. O. Schmitt, R. C. Williams, M. D. Rosenburg and R. H. Bolt. Wiley, New York.

Lemarchand-Béraud, T., Vannotti, A. and Scazziga, B-R. (1967). Plasma TSH levels in the different forms of thyrotoxicosis. In "Thyrotoxicosis". Proceedings of an International Symposium, Edinburgh. Edited by W. J. Irvine, p. 48. Livingstone, Edinburgh.

Lieberthal, A. S., Benson, S. G. and Klitgaard, H. M. (1963). Serum malic dehydrogenase in thyroid disease. *J. clin. Endocr. Metab.*, **23,** 211.

Liechti, H. (1938). Zur Frage der Muskelveränderungen bei Morbus Basedowii. *Endokrinologie*, **20**, 81.

Liu, C-T. and Overman, R. R. (1964). Effect of toxic doses of L-thyroxine on tissue water, electrolytes and plasma protein in rats. *Proc. Soc. exp. Biol. Med.*, **117**, 232.

Logothetis, J. and Warner, J. (1962). Acute thyrotoxic "encephalomyopathy" associated with low serum potassium. *Amer. J. Med.*, **32**, 631.

Loomis, W. F. and Lipmann, F. (1948). Reversible inhibition of the coupling between phosphorylation and oxidation. *J. biol. Chem.*, **173**, 807.

Ludin, H. P., Spiess, H. and Koenig, M. P. (1969). Neuromuscular dysfunction associated with hyperthyroidism. *Europ. Neurol.*, **2**, 269.

Luft, R., Ikkos, D., Palmieri, G., Ernster, L. and Afzelius, B. (1962). A case of severe hypermetabolism of non-thyroid origin with a defect in the maintenance of the mitochondrial respiratory control; a correlated clinical, biochemical and morphological study. *J. clin. Imvest.*, **41**, 1776.

McEachern, D. and Ross, W. D. (1942). Chronic thyrotoxic myopathy: a report of three cases with a review of previously reported cases. *Brain*, **65**, 181.

MacKenzie, M. V. (1940). Chronic thyrotoxic myopathy; report of case complicated with diabetes mellitus. *U.S. Nav. med. Bull.*, **38**, 381.

Malcolm, J. L. and Whitehead, V. I. E. (1944). Muscular fatigue in albino rat and its relationship to thyroid. *Brit. J. exper. Path.*, **25**, 160.

Margreth, A., Salviati, G. and Mussini, I. (1970). The comparative biochemistry of mitochondria and sarcoplasmic reticulum fragments of fast and slow muscle. In "Proceedings of an International Congress on Muscle Diseases". Milan, 1969. Edited by J. N. Walton, N. Canal and G. Scarlato, p. 688. Excerpta Medica, Amsterdam.

Marsden, C. D. and Meadows, J. C. (1970). The effect of adrenaline on the contraction of human muscle. *J. Physiol.* (*Lond.*), **207**, 429.

Massey, D. G., Becklake, M. R., McKenzie, J. M. and Bates, D. V. (1967). Circulatory and ventilatory response to exercise in thyrotoxicosis. *New Engl. J. Med.*, **276**, 1104.

Melville, I. D. (1959). Chronic thyrotoxic myopathy. *Scott. med. J.*, **4**, 318.

Millikan, C. H. and Haines, S. F. (1953). The thyroid gland in relation to neuromuscular disease. *Arch. intern. Med.*, **92**, 5.

Mommaerts, W. F. H. M. (1963). The muscle cell and its functional architecture. *Amer. J. Med.*, **35**, 606.

Morgan, H. J. and Williams, R. H. (1940). Muscular atrophy and weakness in thyrotoxicosis (thyrotoxic myopathy; exophthalmic ophthalmoplegia). *Sth. med. J.* (*Bgham., Ala.*), **33**, 261.

Munro, D. S., Renschler, H. and Wilson, G. M. (1958). Exchangeable potassium and sodium in hyperthyroidism and hypothyroidism. *Metabolism*, **7**, 124.

Namikawa, M. (1970). Studies on calcium and magnesium metabolism. II. Calcium and magnesium in muscle in various neuro-muscular diseases (Jap.). *J. med. Soc. Toho Univ.*, **17,** 50.

Neguib, M. A. (1963). Effect of magnesium on the thyroid. *Lancet*, *i*, 1405.

Norris, F. H. Jr. (1966). Neuromuscular transmission in thyroid disease. *Ann. intern. Med.*, **64,** 81.

Nuttall, F. Q. and Doe, R. P. (1964). The Achilles reflex in thyroid disorders. A critical evaluation. *Ann. intern. Med.*, **61,** 269.

O'Brien, T. W. and Klitgaard, H. M. (1965). Electron microscope study of *in vivo* effects of thyroxine on rat liver mitochondria. *J. Cell Biol.*, **27,** 74A.

Osserman, K. E. and Silver, S. (1961). Advances in Thyroid Research. Edited by R. Pitt-Rivers, p. 100. Pergamon Press, Oxford.

Pace, N. and Rathbun, E. N. (1945). Studies on body composition. III. The body water and chemically combined nitrogen content in relation to fat content. *J. Biol. Chem.*, **158,** 685.

Parsons, F. B. and Twort, R. J. (1939). Chronic thyrotoxic myopathy cured by thyroidectomy. *Lancet*, *i*, 1379.

Paulson, D. L. (1939). Experimental exophthalmos and muscle degeneration induced by thyrotropic hormone. *Proc. Mayo Clin.*, **14,** 828.

Pearce, J. M. S., Pennington, R. J. and Walton, J. N. (1964). Serum enzyme studies in muscle disease. II. Serum creatine kinase activity in muscular dystrophy and in other myopathic and neuropathic disorders. *J. Neurol. Neurosurg. Psychiat.*, **27,** 96.

Pellegrini, G. and Scarlato, G. (1970). Myopathic changes in bilateral exophthalmic ophthalmoplegia. In "Proceedings of an International Congress on Muscle Diseases, Milan, 1969". Edited by J. N. Walton, N. Canal and G. Scarlato, p. 516. Excerpta Medica, Amsterdam.

Peter, J. B., Worsfold, M. and Stempel, K. (1970). Mechanisms of hypermetabolism and of rapid contraction and relaxation of muscle in hyperthyroidism. In "Proceedings of an International Congress on Muscle Diseases. Milan, 1969". Edited by J. N. Walton, N. Canal and G. Scarlato, p. 506. Excerpta Medica, Amsterdam.

Peters, J. H., Schwartz, R., Mermelstein, H., Nefores, M. N. and Mansuy, M. M. (1951). Studies of serum creatine tolerance. I. Findings in normal males and in hyperthyroidism. *J. clin. Invest.*, **30,** 799.

Peterson, R. E. (1958). The influence of the thyroid on adrenal cortical function. *J. clin. Invest.*, **37,** 736.

Pimstone, B. L., Hoffenberg, R. and Black, E. (1963). Parallel assays of thyrotropin, long-acting thyroid stimulator and exophthalmos producing substance in some endocrine disorders. *J. clin. Endocr.*, **23,** 336.

Pimstone, N., Marine, N. and Pimstone, B. (1968). Beta-adrenergic blockade in thyrotoxic myopathy. *Lancet*, *ii*, 1219.

Pinelli, P. and Buchthal, F. (1953). Muscle action potentials in myopathies with special regard to progressive muscular dystrophy. *Neurology* (*Minneap.*), **3,** 347.

Pipberger, H., Kälin, R. and Wegmann, T. (1955). Muskuläre Störungen bei der Hyperthyreose. *Schweiz. med. Wschr.*, **85,** 390.

Plummer, H. S. and Boothby, W. M. (1923). The cost of work in exophthalmic goiter. *Amer. J. Physiol.*, **63,** 406.

Price, H. M. (1969). In "Disorders of Voluntary Muscle". Edited by J. N. Walton, p. 29. Churchill, London.

Quinn, E. L. and Worcester, R. L. (1951). Chronic thyrotoxic myopathy; report of a case. *J. clin. Endocr.*, **11,** 1564.

Ramsay, I. D. (1964). The muscle lesion in thyrotoxicosis. M.D. Thesis, University of Edinburgh.

Ramsay, I. D. (1965). Electromyography in thyrotoxicosis. *Quart. J. Med.*, **34,** 255.

Ramsay, I. D. (1966). Muscle dysfunction in hyperthyroidism. *Lancet*, *ii*, 931.

Ramsay, I. D. (1970). Unpublished.

Ramsay, I., Marsden, P., Richardson, P. J. and McKerron, C. G. (1972). Thyroid "hot" nodules. *Postgrad. med. J.*, **48,** 577.

Ringqvist, I. (1970). Achilles reflex time as a measure of thyroid function. *Acta med. scand.*, **188,** 231.

Robison, G. A., Butcher, R. W. and Sutherland, E. W. (1967). Adenyl cyclase as an adrenergic receptor. *Ann. N.Y. Acad. Sci.*, **139,** 703.

Rosenbaum, E. E., Portis, S. and Soskin, S. (1941). The relief of muscular weakness by pyridoxine hydrochloride. *J. lab. clin. Med.*, **27,** 763.

Sacco, G., Buchthal, F. and Rosenfalck, P. (1962). Motor unit potentials at different ages. *Arch. Neurol.* (*Chic.*), **6,** 366.

Sacrez, R., Lausecker, C. and Isch, C. (1955). Association de maladie de Basedow, de myopathie et de tetanie chez une enfant de 11 ans. *Arch. franç. Pédiat.*, **12,** 944.

Sanderson, K. V. and Adey, W. R. (1949). Chronic thyrotoxic myopathy, with report of case including electromyographic studies. *Med. J. Aust.*, *i*, 797.

Sanderson, K. V. and Adey, W. R. (1952). Electromyographic and endocrine studies in chronic thyrotoxic myopathy. *J. Neurol. Neurosurg. Psychiat.*, **15,** 200.

Sanghvi, L. M., Gupta, K. D., Banerjee, K. and Bose, K. (1959). Paraplegia, hypokalaemia and nephropathy with muscle lesions of potassium deficiency associated with thyrotoxicosis. *Amer. J. Med.*, **27,** 817.

Satoyoshi, E., Murakami, K., Kowa, H., Kinoshita, M., Noguchi, K., Hoshina, S., Nishiyama, Y. and Ito, K. (1963a). Myopathy in thyrotoxicosis, with special emphasis on an effect of potassium ingestion on serum and urinary creatine. *Neurology* (*Minneap.*), **13,** 645.

Satoyoshi, E., Murakami, K. and Torii, J. (1963b). Thyrotoxic myopathy. *Lancet*, *ii*, 843.

Sattler, H. (1952). "Basedow's Disease". (English translation by G. W. and J. F. Marchand.) Grune and Stratton, New York.

Schwartz, N. B., Ingold, A. H., Hammond, G. E. and Gronert, G. A. (1960). Role of temperature in determining effects of thyroxine and propylthiouracil on the motor unit. *Amer. J. Physiol.*, **198,** 456.

Schwartz, N. B. and Lein, A. (1955). Effects of thyroxin on skeletal muscle function. *Amer. J. Physiol.*, **182,** 5.

Sharpe, A. R. (1961). A simple isotope method for recording the Achilles tendon reflex in myxedema. *J. lab. clin. Med.*, **57,** 165.

Sheldon, J. H. and Walker, R. M. (1946). Acute thyrotoxic myopathy; recovery after partial thyroidectomy. *Lancet*, *i*, 342.

Shishiba, Y., Shizume, K., Sakuma, M., Yamauchi, H., Nakao, K. and Okinaka, S. (1966). Studies on electrolyte metabolism in idiopathic and thyrotoxic periodic paralysis. III. Intra- and extracellular concentrations of potassium and sodium in muscle and their changes during induced attacks of paralysis. *Metabolism*, **15,** 153.

Shizume, K., Shishiba, Y., Sakuma, M., Yamauchi, H., Nakao, K. and Okinaka, S. (1966). Studies on electrolyte metabolism in idiopathic and thyrotoxic periodic paralysis. II. Total exchangeable sodium and potassium. *Metabolism*, **15,** 145.

Shy, G. M., Gonatas, N. K. and Perez, M. (1966). Two childhood myopathies with abnormal mitochondria. I. Megaconial myopathy. II. Pleoconial myopathy. *Brain*, **89,** 133.

Sissons, H. A. (1969). In "Disorders of Voluntary Muscle". Edited by J. N. Walton, p. 1. J. & A. Churchill, London.

Smith, R. E. (1964). Thermogenesis and thyroid action. *Nature*, **204,** 1311.

Smith, R. E. and Whalen, W. J. (1960). Effect of thyroxine on contractile efficiency of rat diaphragm. *Fed. Proc.*, **19,** 175.

Spiro, A. J., Prineas, J. W. and Moore, C. L. (1970). A new mitochondrial myopathy in a patient with salt craving. *Arch. Neurol.*, **22,** 259.

Staffurth, J. S. (1962). Total exchangeable potassium in hyperthyroidism. *Metabolism*, **11,** 1274.

Staffurth, J. S. and Thompson, J. C. (1965). Muscle potassium in thyrotoxicosis. *Metabolism*, **14,** 241.

Starling, H. J., Darke, C. S., Hunt, B. W. and Brain, W. R. (1938). Two cases of Graves' disease with muscular atrophy. *Guy's Hosp. Rep.*, **88,** 117.

Stocker, W. W., Samaha, F. J. and De Groot, L. J. (1968). Coupled oxidative phosphorylation in muscle of thyrotoxic patients. *Amer. J. Med.*, **44,** 900.

Strong, J. A. (1949). Thyrotoxicosis with ophthalmoplegia, myopathy, Wolff-Parkinson-White syndrome and pericardial friction. *Lancet*, *i*, 959.

Tapley, D. F. (1964). Mode and site of action of thyroxine. *Mayo Clin Proc.*, **39,** 626.

Thomas, P. K. (1963). In "Clinical Physiology". Edited by E. J. M. Campbell, C. J. Dickinson and J. D. H. Slater, p. 315. Blackwell Scientific Publications, Oxford.

Thorn, G. W. and Eder, H. A. (1946). Studies on chronic thyrotoxic myopathy. *Amer. J. Med.*, **1,** 583.

Tsujihata, M. (1969). Electron microscopic study of neuromuscular diseases (Jap.). *Clin. Neurol.* (*Tokyo*), **9,** 451.

Van Wijngaarden, G. K., Bethlem, J., Meijer, A. E. F. H., Hülsmann, W-C. and Feltkamp, C. A. (1967). Skeletal muscle disease with abnormal mitochondria. *Brain*, **90,** 577.

Vilppula and Buchthal. (Unpublished), quoted by Buchthal, F. (1970).

Waal-Manning, H. J. (1969). Effect of propranolol on the duration of the Achilles tendon reflex. *Clin. Pharmacol. Ther.*, **10,** 199.

Wachstein, M. and Lobel, S. (1956). The relation between tryptophane metabolism and Vitamin B6 in various diseases as studied by paper chromatography. *Ann. J. clin. Path.*, **26,** 910.

Waldenström, J. (1945). Acute thyrotoxic encephalo- or myopathy, its cause and treatment. *Acta med. scand.*, **121,** 251.

Wang, E. (1939). Clinical and experimental investigations on the creatine metabolism. *Acta med. scand. Supp.* 105.

Wayne, E. J. (1960). Clinical and metabolic studies in thyroid disease. *Brit. med. J.*, *i*, 78.

Whitfield, A. G. W. and Hudson, W. A. (1961). Chronic thyrotoxic myopathy. *Quart. J. Med.*, **30,** 257.

Wilder, V. M. and Morgulis, S. (1953). Creatinuria in normal males. *Arch. Biochem. Biophys.*, **42,** 69.

Wilkins, L. and Fleischmann, W. (1946). Effects of thyroid on creatine metabolism with a discussion of the mechanism of storage and excretion of creatine bodies. *J. clin. Invest.*, **25,** 360.

Wohl, M. G., Levy, H. A., Szutka, A. and Maldia, G. (1960). Pyridoxine deficiency in hyperthyroidism. *Proc. Soc. exp. Biol. Med.*, **105,** 523.

Yates, D. A. H. (1963). The estimation of mean potential duration in endocrine myopathy. *J. Neurol. Neurosurg. Psychiat.*, **26,** 458.

Yates, D. A. H. (1965). Electrodiagnosis of myopathic disorders. *Postgrad. med. J.*, **41,** 325.

Zaimis, E., Metaxas, N., Havard, C. W. H. and Campbell, E. D. R. (1965). Cardiovascular and skeletal muscle changes in cats treated with thyroxine. In "Research in Muscular Dystrophy". Edited by members of the Research Committee of the Muscular Dystrophy Group, p. 301. Pitman Medical, London.

Zaimis, E., Papadaki, L., Kakari, S., Mathew, M., Ash, A. S. F., Larbi, E. and Paradelis, A. (1968). Mitochondrial and Myofibrillar changes in Induced Myopathies. In "Research in Muscular Dystrophy". Edited by members of the Research Committee of the Muscular Dystrophy Group, p. 395. Pitman Medical, London.

Zierler, K. L. (1951). Muscle wasting of obscure origin and the thyroid gland. *Bull. Johns Hopk. Hosp.*, **89,** 263.

Zierler, K. L. (1970). Diseases of Muscle in "Biochemical Disorders in Human Disease". Edited by R. H. S. Thompson and I. D. P. Wootton, p. 489. Churchill, London.

CHAPTER 2

THYROID DISEASE AND MYASTHENIA GRAVIS

In 1908 Rennie described a patient with both exophthalmic goitre and myasthenia gravis. He regarded them as coincidental, but since then a steadily growing number of similar reports has indicated that there appears to be more than a chance association between the two diseases. More recently it has been suggested that hypothyroidism may occur in conjunction with myasthenia gravis just as commonly as thyrotoxicosis, if not more so (Sahay, Blendis and Greene, 1965). Simpson (1968) claimed that thyroid disease of one sort or other was present in 18% of his series of 518 myasthenic patients. Since 1960 interest has been centred on myasthenia gravis (Simpson, 1960), Graves' disease, Hashimoto's thyroiditis and primary hypothyroidism as being examples of autoimmune disease (Anderson *et al.*, 1964; Roitt and Doniach, 1960). It would seem important therefore to examine the relationship between thyroid disease and myasthenia gravis in order to determine whether there are common causative factors and to discover what effects variation in thyroid hormone status has upon myasthenia gravis.

THYROTOXICOSIS AND MYASTHENIA GRAVIS

Prevalence

Myasthenia gravis is a fairly rare disease. Pennington and Wilson (1961) in a survey of the Merseyside conurbation found an overall prevalence* of 1 in 43,343 of the general population, which was in good agreement with an earlier figure of 1 in 40,000 derived by Garland and Clark (1956) in Yorkshire. Pennington and Wilson found a 1·5:1 female to male ratio which is similar to the ratio of 2·1:1 found in J. A. Simpson's (1968) series of 518 myasthenic patients and to the ratio of 1·4:1 in the 295 patients of J. F. Simpson and his colleagues (1966).

Thyrotoxicosis, on the other hand, is a much more common disease. Population figures are hard to come by as it is not a

* Prevalence: the number of cases existing in a population at any given time.

notifiable disease and, since the advent of antithyroid drugs and radioactive iodine treatment, a majority of patients are not admitted to hospital. Nevertheless, Iversen (1948) calculated that in the city of Copenhagen in the years before the Second World War the incidence* of thyrotoxicosis was 0·2 per 1000 of the general population. Logan and Cushion (1958), examining morbidity statistics for general practice in England and Wales for the year 1955–56 found an incidence of 1·1 per 1000 of the population, or 0·3 per 1000 men and 1·9 per 1000 women, giving roughly a 6 to 1 female to male ratio. These figures for the incidence of thrytoxicosis are rather higher than Iversen's but this may reflect the development of more sophisticated diagnostic techniques.

TABLE 2.1

Prevalence of myasthenia gravis in thyrotoxic patients

Authors	Number of thyrotoxics	Number of thyrotoxics with myasthenia gravis	Prevalence of myasthenia gravis %
Bartels and Kingsley (1949)	12,962	4	0·03
Osserman and Silver (1961)	4,000	14	0·35
Sahay *et al.* (1965)	$>$12,000	3	c. 0·025
Simpson (1968)	1,019	2	0·20
Total	c. 29,945	23	0·08

Myasthenia gravis is said to be a rare complication of thyrotoxicosis (Simpson, 1968). Table 2.1 summarizes the prevalence of myasthenia gravis in patients with thyrotoxicosis. Out of nearly 30,000 thyrotoxic patients, 23 had myasthenia gravis, giving a prevalence rate of 0·77 per 1000. However, this figure is 30 times greater than the prevalence of myasthenia gravis in the general population. If one looks at the prevalence of thyrotoxicosis in patients with myasthenia gravis (Table 2.2) it can be seen that 5% of over 3500 myasthenic patients developed thyrotoxicosis (50 per 1000). Bearing in mind the inherent errors in both population and

* Incidence: the number of cases occurring per unit of population within a defined time interval (usually a year).

TABLE 2.2

Prevalence of thyrotoxicosis in patients with myasthenia gravis

Authors	Number of myasthenics	Number of thyrotoxics	Prevalence of thyrotoxicosis %
Bartels and Kingsley (1949)	90	4	4·4
Grob and Harvey (1953)	270	8	3·0
Millikan and Haines (1953)	500	25	5·0
Oosterhuis (1964)	180	8	4·4
Sahay *et al.* (1965)	260	3	1·2
Rowland *et al.* (1966)	400	20	5·0
Schimrick (1966)	70	7	10·0
Simpson, J. F. *et al.* (1966)	295	24	8·1
Wolf *et al.* (1966)	399	22	5·5
Osserman *et al.* (1967)	801	42	5·2
Simpson, J. A. (1968)	518	37	7·1
Kotlyarov *et al.* (1969)	172	6	3·5
Total	3,955	206	5·2

clinical surveys and the difficulty in comparing figures for prevalence and incidence, there appears to be an increase in both the prevalence of myasthenia in thyrotoxics and in the prevalence of thyrotoxicosis in myasthenics. It suggests that there is a very definite link between the two diseases. It has already been noted that in the general population, women develop thyrotoxicosis six times as frequently as men. Similarly, as can be seen from Table 2.3, female myasthenics become thyrotoxic between two and five times as commonly as men.

The mean age of onset of myasthenia gravis is at 26 years for women and 30 for men (Brain and Walton, 1969). Similarly, Graves' disease is said to be most common between the age of 20 and 40 (Means, De Groot and Stanbury, 1963). This may be additional tentative evidence supporting a causative link between the two diseases. Just as thyrotoxicosis is a rare disease in children, so is the combination of the disease with myasthenia gravis. Schlezinger and Corin described in 1968 only the seventh case in the world literature. Of the patients 5 were girls and 2 were boys. In only 4 of the 7 cases did the myasthenia present before the age of 15. In 5 of the 7 cases myasthenia gravis developed after the onset of thyrotoxicosis at intervals varying from three months to 20 years.

The frequency with which hyperthyroidism occurs in myasthenia

TABLE 2.3

The prevalence of thyrotoxicosis in female and male patients with myasthenia gravis

Authors	Female patients			Male patients		
	Number of myasthenics	Number with thyrotoxicosis	%	Number of myasthenics	Number with thyrotoxicosis	%
Simpson, J. F., *et al*. (1966)	171	21	12·3	124	3	2·4
Simpson, J. A. (1968)	351	30	8·5	167	7	4·2
Totals	522	51	9·8	291	10	3·4

may be even higher than the 5·0% suggested in Table 2.2. Simpson (1968), in a series of 66 patients in whom a systematic study of thyroid function was made, found 3 cases of clinical hyperthyroidism and 3 patients in whom the disease was only discovered as the result of the investigations. This is a prevalence of 9%. The association may be even more striking if one considers patients with severe myasthenia. Glaser (1966) found 4 patients with hyperthyroidism out of 20 who were either in acute myasthenic crisis or were resistant to anticholinesterase drugs, representing a prevalence of 20%.

Temporal relationships. There seems little doubt from the evidence which has been presented that there is a close relationship between thyrotoxicosis and myasthenia gravis. It is important to examine the true relationship between the onset of the two diseases. Table 2.4 shows data from original studies (Millikan and Haines, 1953, Rowland

TABLE 2.4

Showing the time relationship between the two diseases in patients with both thyrotoxicosis and myasthenia gravis

Authors	Millikan and Haines (1953) %	Engel (1961) %	Rowland *et al.* (1966) %	Kissel *et al.* (1970) %
Thyrotoxicosis first	48	76 (thyrotoxicosis first and simultaneous combined)	50	45
Simultaneous	20		30	20–25
Myasthenia gravis first	32		20	30–35

et al., 1966) and from reviews of the literature by Engel (1961) and by Kissel *et al.* (1970). There is good agreement among these three sources, in that 30–35% of patients developed myasthenia gravis first, 45–48% developed thyrotoxicosis as the first disease and in 20–25% of patients the two diseases occurred concurrently. Engel (1961) did not give separate figures for the three groups but noted that in 76% of cases the thyrotoxicosis occurred before or at the same time as the myasthenia. Millikan and Haines (1953) noted that in a quarter of their patients who got thyrotoxicosis first, the disease anticipated the onset of myasthenia by more than five years.

Simpson's (1968) experience was similar in 37 thyrotoxic myasthenic patients. Bearing in mind the above relationships, it is obvious that in some patients the thyrotoxicosis will be subsiding or be in complete remission as the myasthenia develops and that in others the myasthenia is remitting as thyrotoxicosis appears. This relationship has been blessed with the title of "see-saw" (McEachern and Parnell, 1948) and is always quoted in works on the subject. In fact, the "see-saw" relationship between thyrotoxicosis and myasthenia gravis has been supported in a minority of reports (Thorner, 1939; Cohen, 1946; Maclean and Wilson, 1954) and most authors conclude that the two diseases evolve in parallel or show no very obvious clinical pattern of interaction (Thorn and Tierney, 1941; Kowallis, Haines and Pemberton, 1942; Flynn, 1944; Greene, 1949; Millikan and Haines, 1953; Osserman and Silver, 1961). Kissel and his colleagues (1965) in their review of all the cases published up to that time, came to the conclusion that exacerbations of the thyrotoxicosis caused worsening of the myasthenia and that remission of the hyperthyroidism brought about improvement of the myasthenia ("evolutive parallelism") in 40%; that myasthenia improved with the onset of thyrotoxicosis and became more severe when the thyrotoxicosis remitted ("evolutive antagonism") in 20%; and that there was no reciprocal influence in 15% of cases. The relationship was unclear or undetermined in 25%.

It thus seems that the commonest circumstance is for the thyrotoxicosis to have an adverse effect on the myasthenia. This would fit in with the impression that thyrotoxic myasthenia has a worse prognosis than myasthenia gravis alone (Millikan and Haines, 1953; Glaser, 1966) and with the studies of Engel (1961) and Drachman (1962). Engel (1961) studied the effect of administering triiodothyronine to 5 euthyroid patients with myasthenia gravis. Moderate doses of the hormone, sufficient to block the pituitary release of thyroid stimulating hormone (TSH), but not enough to raise the basal metabolic rate, had no effect on the myasthenia. Larger doses, producing hypermetabolism, aggravated the myasthenia. When hypermetabolism was produced by giving exogenous TSH it had a similar result, but when the effect of TSH on the release of hormone from the thyroid gland was blocked by sodium iodide, the TSH administration did not influence the myasthenic state adversely. Engel thus concluded that TSH itself had no effect on myasthenic weakness but that excess exogenous or endogenous thyroid hormone made it worse. Drachman (1962) gave varying doses of triiodothyronine to a patient with both myasthenia and myxoedema. The myasthenia, which was minimal when the patient was euthyroid, became worse when hyperthyroidism was induced.

One must conclude that there is no clear and simple link between thyrotoxicosis and myasthenia gravis. The parallel development of the two diseases seems to be the commonest and excess thyroid hormone frequently causes an exacerbation of the myasthenia, but it can be seen from the above data that there are many exceptions to the rule.

Genetic factors. Namba and his colleagues recently reported that 3·8% of 702 patients with myasthenia gravis had a positive family history for the disease (Namba *et al.*, 1971). They concluded that, since the most common familial occurrence of the disease was in siblings, the most likely mode of inheritance was autosomal recessive.

In a study of 204 patients with Graves' disease in Copenhagen, Bartels (1941) found that there was a positive family history in 60% and thought it likely that the inheritance was autosomal recessive with a relative sex limitation to women and a penetrance of 70–80%.

It is possible that a similar type of inheritance of two diseases which are thought to have an auto-immune basis may be the linking factor.

Clinical presentation.—The clinical picture will obviously depend on the sequence in which thyrotoxicosis and myasthenia gravis occur and the severity with which each presents. In the commonest situation the thyrotoxicosis will have been present already, and may even be in remission, when the symptoms of myasthenia appear *de novo*. In this particular case the diagnosis should not be too difficult as the clinical picture does not differ from that found in pure myasthenia. The patient typically complains of ptosis or diplopia which either develops or gets worse towards the end of the day. In more severe cases the patient may have difficulty in swallowing or chewing towards the end of a meal. In other cases the patient notices fatigue of the limbs which is more marked in the proximal than in the distal muscles. Finally, the muscles of the trunk and of respiration are affected. Table 2.5 shows the spread of muscle involvement in 220 cases of myasthenia gravis. This pattern of involvement is quite different from that seen in thyrotoxic patients with muscle weakness, but without myasthenia gravis, in whom the proximal muscles of the upper and lower limbs are most commonly affected, distal muscles of the limbs less so and muscles of the trunk, neck and face hardly at all (Havard *et al.*, 1963; Ramsay, 1966).

TABLE 2.5

Showing the different patterns and sequence of muscle involvement in myasthenia gravis and in thyrotoxicosis

Pattern of muscle involvement in myasthenia gravis*	Pattern of muscle involvement in thyrotoxicosis†
Extraocular muscles	Upper limbs: proximal muscles
Orbicularis oculi	
Frontalis	Lower limbs: proximal muscles
Orbicularis oris	
Swallowing	
Speech	
Mastication	
Tongue	
Upper limbs: proximal > distal	Distal limb muscles
Lower limbs: proximal > distal	
Trunk	
Abdomen	
Respiration	Bulbar muscles

* Grob and Harvey (1953). † Ramsay (1966, 1968).

However, in patients described in the literature as having "chronic thyrotoxic myopathy", 16·4% had evidence of bulbar muscle paresis (Ramsay, 1964) and a recent paper from Australia (Joasoo, Murray and Steinbeck, 1970) suggests that bulbar muscle involvement in uncomplicated thyrotoxicosis may be more frequent than was previously thought.

An additional problem is the occurrence of myasthenia gravis in a thyrotoxic patient who has exophthalmos. Of the 20 patients with

TABLE 2.6

Ocular signs in patients with myasthenia gravis and thyrotoxicosis (Rowland, Aranow and Hoefer, 1966)

	Number of patients
Thyrotoxicosis and myasthenia gravis	20
Distribution of weakness: eyes alone	10
generalized	10
Ocular signs: ptosis and exophthalmos	12
ptosis alone	7
exophthalmos alone	1

thyrotoxicosis and myasthenia gravis reported from the Columbia-Presbyterian Medical Center by Rowland and his colleagues, 12 patients had "some degree of exophthalmos" though the authors did not define their terms (Rowland, Aranow and Hoefer, 1966). Details of the patients are given in Table 2.6. It can be seen that in half the patients weakness was confined to the eye muscles while in the other half the weakness was generalized. Ptosis, even in the presence of exophthalmos, was almost a constant feature. All of the patients had a good response to edrophonium or neostigmine. The changes of "infiltrative ophthalmopathy" were seen in 3 patients and, in one of them, were bad enough to be called "malignant exophthalmos". This patient required orbital decompression. Over a ten-year period his eye condition settled, but he was left with residual exophthalmos and ocular muscle weakness which responded to edrophonium. It is suggested that the extra-ocular muscle weakness may have been due to a combination of myasthenia and malignant infiltrative disease.

It is, of course, not necessary for the myasthenia gravis and exophthalmos to be associated with the hyperthyroid state. Of Grob and Harvey's (1953) 270 patients with myasthenia, 6 had exophthalmos in the absence of any current or previous thyroid disease. This situation is well recognized in thyroid clinics (Werner, 1955).

It is in the patient who presents with a possible combination of thyrotoxicosis and myasthenia gravis that the greatest difficulty lies, for one has to decide whether the patient is suffering from thyrotoxic myopathy with bulbar involvement plus infiltrative ophthalmopathy or whether the patient has predominantly myasthenia gravis with bulbar and ocular involvement and associated wasting and weakness of proximal limb muscles. The following case history illustrates some of these features.

Case R.V.H. 684023. She was a 35-year-old Northern Irish housewife who presented at the Royal Victoria Hospital, Belfast, in May 1963 with a three months' history of light-headedness, palpitations and a weight loss of 32 lb. (14·5 kg). For two weeks she had noticed drooping of the left eyelid and some diplopia from about 11 o'clock in the morning onwards, which was not present on rising in the morning. She denied any other muscle symptoms. On examination she was a thin, nervous woman (Fig. 2.1). Her pulse was 112 per minute and in sinus rhythm. Her hands were hot and sweaty and she had marked finger tremor. Her thyroid gland was only slightly enlarged (30 G); it was smooth and a bruit was present. She had marked wasting of the supraspinati, infraspinati, triceps, biceps, glutei and temporalis muscles and a lesser degree of wasting of her deltoids (Fig. 2.1). There was pronounced weakness of the supraspinatus, infraspinatus and triceps on both sides, and slightly less weakness of the deltoids, biceps, glutei, iliopsoas and wrist extensor muscles. Using the modified Lahey test (Ramsay, 1966), the patient was able to keep her legs elevated at 45° for an average of 25 sec.

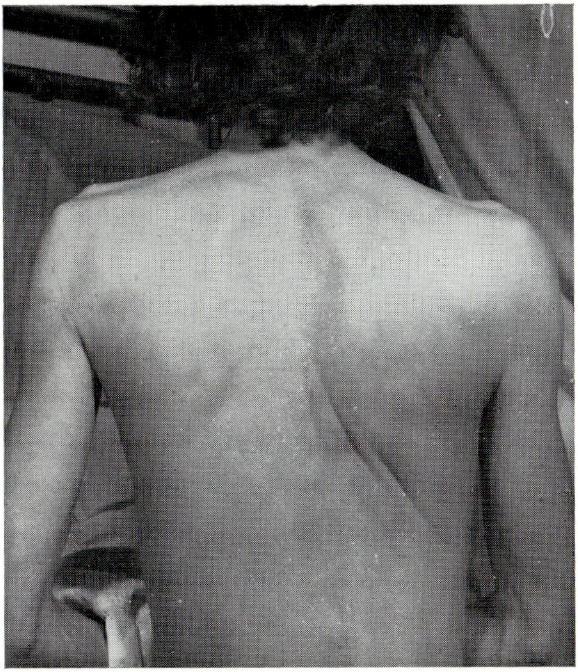

Figure 2.1. Thirty-five-year-old female patient with thyrotoxicosis and myasthenia gravis; showing wasting of the shoulder girdle muscles.

only. The lower limit of normal is 77 sec. (Ramsay, 1967). There was no fasciculation. She had no exophthalmos (Hertel exophthalmometer readings 13 mm for right eye, 12 mm for left eye), but had bilateral ptosis (Fig. 2.2a), worse on the left. She had diplopia in all directions of gaze caused by involvement of all the extraocular muscles of the left eye and the lateral and medial rectus muscles of the right eye (Fig. 2.2b). She was given 10 mg of edrophonium

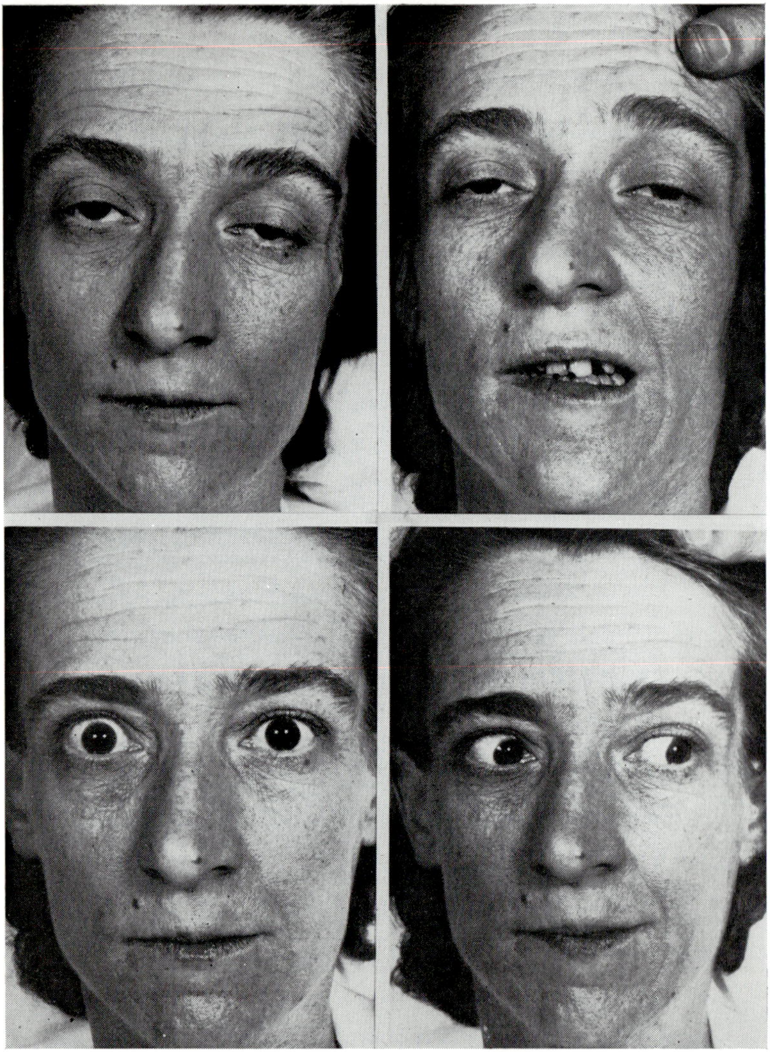

(*a*) (*b*)

(*c*) (*d*)

Figure 2.1. The same patient as in Fig. 2.1, showing (*a*) ptosis, (*b*) attempts to look to the left, (*c*) lid retraction after the injection of edrophonium and (*d*) partial recovery of extraocular muscle function following edrophonium.

chloride (Tensilon) intravenously. This produced no increase in muscle power and Lahey's modified test was only improved to 32 sec. The effect on the eyes, however, was dramatic (Fig. 2.2c, d). Her ptosis disappeared and she demonstrated lid retraction. Her extra-ocular muscle paresis improved considerably, though she still had some double vision on downward gaze and to the left. An electro-myogram of the deltoid done without the influence of edrophonium showed clear-cut evidence of a myopathy with a mean action potential duration of 6·7 m sec. (predicted for age 11·4 m sec.), 27% polyphasic potentials and an interference pattern on maximal effort. No insertional activity was found, and there was no evidence of denervation or of fasciculation. Supramaximal stimulation of the ulnar nerve produced no fatigue of the muscle action potentials and there was no change in this amplitude after the same stimulation following the injection of edrophonium.

The diagnosis of thyrotoxicosis was confirmed by a P.B.I. of 13·2 μg % and an ^{131}I T_3 red cell uptake of 39.4%. Her 24-hour urinary creatine was 330 mg and creatinine 770 mg.

Two days after her first visit she was started on carbimazole 20 mg q.i.d. Four and a half weeks later she had put on 9 lb. (4 kg) in weight and her muscle power had returned to normal. The girth of her thighs had increased by 1·25 inches (3·1 cm). Her ptosis had disappeared but she still had diplopia to right and left and on downward gaze. L-Thyroxine 0·2 mg per day was added into her regime. When she was admitted for partial thyroidectomy five months after her initial presentation she had put on 16 lb. (7·2 kg) in weight, had no evidence of muscle wasting (thigh circumference 2 inches (5 cm) greater than originally) and could produce a 120-second result for the modified Lahey test. However, she had some ptosis of the right eye and had diplopia on looking to the left and on upward gaze.

Two weeks after partial thyroidectomy her diplopia improved dramatically. When she was reviewed six years later in 1969 she was found to be euthyroid, with no exophthalmos (Hertel: right eye 14 mm, left eye 14 mm) and no clinically evident diplopia, though she did say that occasionally she got slight double vision when she was tired.

This case shows that myasthenia gravis and thyrotoxic myopathy can exist coincidentally and independently in the same patient. The myasthenia gravis appears to have been confined to the extraocular muscles, for edrophonium had no effect on either increasing muscle power in the proximal limb muscles or in altering the response to tetanic stimulation. After four and a half weeks of treatment with antithyroid drugs her muscle power had returned to normal and by five months all evidence of proximal wasting had disappeared, yet she still had symptoms referable to ocular myasthenia gravis. This itself improved dramatically following partial thyroidectomy and over a six-year period. She only occasionally had minimal diplopia attributable to myasthenia gravis. It is interesting to speculate why it was that the myasthenia improved so rapidly two weeks after subtotal thyroidectomy. Was it merely coincidental, or could it in some way have been related to the removal of the thyroid antigen to which Long Acting Thyroid Stimulator is an antibody? A study of the degree of remission of myasthenia gravis produced by the treatment of co-existing thyrotoxicosis by surgery as compared with antithyroid drugs might be rewarding.

Diagnosis. Clinically the differentiation between myasthenia gravis with hyperthyroidism and pure thyrotoxic myopathy is fairly straightforward. The more prominent symptoms of the patient with myasthenia gravis will be ptosis, diplopia, dysarthria and dysphagia, there will be a variation in the degree of weakness throughout the day and a worsening with repetitive activity. The patient with myopathy, on the other hand, will have complaints associated mainly with proximal muscle weakness. Only occasionally will bulbar muscles be involved and it is in these patients that careful investigation to exclude myasthenia gravis must be performed. It would, for instance, be dangerous to perform a partial thyroidectomy on any patient with bulbar myasthenia gravis unless this had been absolutely controlled by appropriate therapy.

Investigations

Edrophonium (Tensilon) test. The simplest test to perform is the injection of 10 mg of edrophonium chloride (Tensilon) intravenously. Initially 2 mg is injected to detect abnormal sensitivity. If no response appears after 30 seconds the remaining 8 mg is given (Osserman and Kaplan, 1953). If the weakness improves within one minute and relapses four or five minutes later, the test indicates myasthenia gravis. Thyrotoxic muscle weakness does not respond to edrophonium (Ramsay, 1966) but it is important when assessing this to use an objective test of muscle weakness. A simple one is a modification of Lahey's (1926) test in which the patient lies on a bed and, with the leg straight, raises it to an angle of 45 degrees and keeps it there as long as possible. The 95% confidence limit for the lower extreme of normal is 77 seconds (Ramsay, 1967).

As an alternative to edrophonium, neostigmine methylsulphate (Prostigmin) 1·5 mg may be injected intramuscularly combined with 0·6 mg of atropine sulphate to prevent any adverse effect on the heart. The response begins in 10–15 minutes and is complete by about 30 minutes. The test does have one advantage over the edrophonium test in that the investigator does have more time to examine the affected muscle groups (Viets and Schwab, 1935).

In the case of edrophonium, following the injection subjects may feel periorbital tightness and fasciculation of the orbicularis oculi may be found.

Prostigmin or edrophonium was given to 27 of the cases of "chronic thyrotoxic myopathy" described in the literature (Ramsay, 1968). No increase in power was noticed in 24 instances and it produced a good response in only one patient (McEachern and Ross, 1942) and a slight response in a further two (Sanderson and Adey, 1952; Melville, 1959). Havard *et al.* (1963) assessed muscular strength in 49 thyrotoxics before and 30 minutes after 1·5 mg of intramuscular neostigmine. Forty-three patients showed no increase in power, but 6 were thought to be stronger, though the authors do not give any statistical data. Ramsay (1966) found no difference in the length of time for which 19 unselected thyrotoxics could perform the modified Lahey test before and after edrophonium.

If there is still doubt about the diagnosis of myasthenia gravis after the performance of the edrophonium or neostigmine tests the following tests are helpful.

D-Tubocurarine

The curarizing dose for a normal adult is 3 mg of d-tubocurarine intravenously per 40 lb. body weight (Simpson, 1969). Patients with myasthenia gravis become weak with 5% or less of the curarizing dose, whereas the weakness of hyperthyroid patients with myopathy is not made worse.

Decamethonium

Churchill-Davidson and Richardson (1952) showed that myasthenics are much more resistant to the action of decamethonium than normals. Decamethonium iodide is injected intravenously in a dosage of 0·5 mg per minute, up to a maximum of 3 mg. This will produce extreme weakness or paralysis in the normal subject or the ordinary thyrotoxic patient, but will probably not do so in the patient with myasthenia gravis. It should be noted that when weakness does occur in the myasthenic patient, it affects first of all the muscles which are clinically involved, so facilities for resuscitation should be immediately available. The paresis in the myasthenic patient is reversible by edrophonium, but this has no effect on the normal subject or the patient with thyrotoxicosis (Osserman and Silver, 1961).

Electromyography

Since the electromyographic finding of a myopathy is an almost constant feature of thyrotoxicosis (see Chapter 1, p. 9) the E.M.G. done on minimal effort will be of little help in the thyrotoxic patient with suspected myasthenia gravis. Moreover, some patients with ocular myasthenia gravis, who do not have thyrotoxicosis, have E.M.G. evidence of a myopathy in extra-ocular muscles (Faurschou, 1970). However, the pattern of electrical activity recorded at maximal effort in a myasthenic patient differs from that of the normal or of the thyrotoxic subject. Maintenance of the effort results in a reduc-

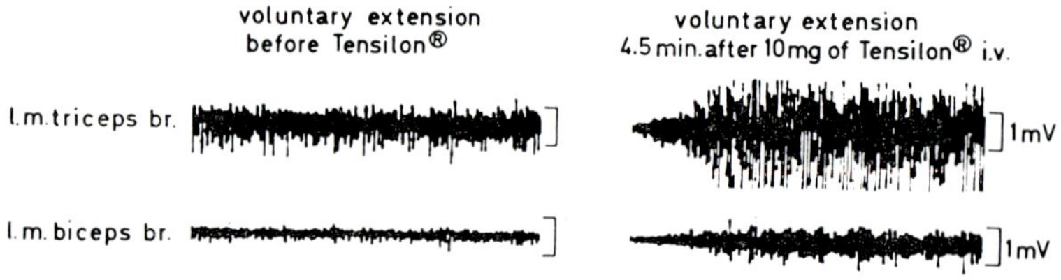

Figure 2.3. Maximum voluntary extension in a myasthenic patient showing the increase in amplitude of the discharge pattern following the administration of edrophonium (Tensilon). (Modified from Buchthal, 1970).

tion in amplitude of the interference pattern and when the muscle is fatigued only a few motor units continue to produce potentials irregularly. This fall off in amplitude and rapid fatiguability of motor unit activity can be reversed by administering edrophonium or prostigmin (Fig. 2.3). However, the alterations in the discharge pattern on voluntary effort before and after edrophonium or prostigmin can be difficult to interpret in skeletal muscles (Slomić, Rosenfalck and Buchthal, 1968), and is best done in the extra-ocular muscles (Faurschou, 1970); though it is possible that this test might not find favour with all patients!

An alternative method of investigating the suspected myasthenic patient is by recording the muscle action potentials and mechanical responses produced by repetitive supramaximal stimulation of the nerve. The technique can be applied to proximal muscles as well as distal, though recordings are often taken from the adductor pollicis muscle with stimulation of the ulnar nerve. This can be done at a frequency of between three and 20 per second and the amplitude of the evoked response recorded on the E.M.G. over a period of a few seconds. Figure 2.4 shows the decline in the action potential amplitude in a patient with myasthenia gravis and its recovery after the administration of edrophonium (Tensilon). The mechanical response produced by the muscle can also be recorded.

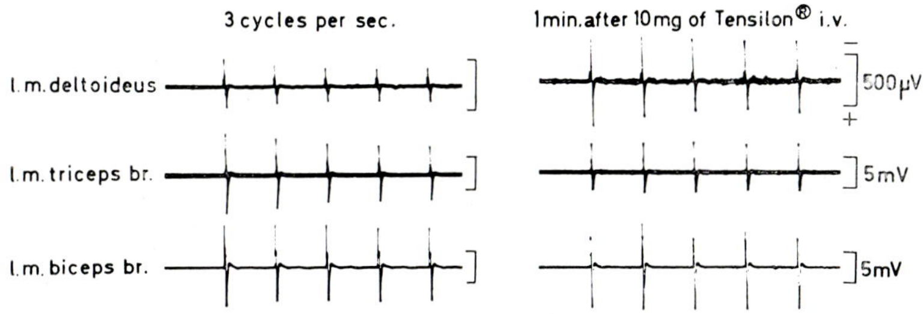

Figure 2.4. Action potentials in a myasthenic patient evoked by supramaximal stimuli to the brachial plexus at 3/sec for 1½ seconds. The amplitude of the discharge in the deltoid and triceps muscles was diminished by 30% and in the biceps by 10%. After 10 mg of edrophonium (Tensilon) intravenously the decrease in the deltoid response was 14% and there was no longer a decrease in the brachial biceps and triceps muscles. (From Buchthal, 1970).

However, Buchthal (1970) has recently pointed out some of the pitfalls of even the supramaximal stimulation technique, particularly when the myasthenia is mild. Distal muscles are least involved clinically, yet it is in these that the procedure is often done. He shows an example of one patient with a myasthenic reaction in proximal muscles, but a normal reaction in a distal muscle. He also remarks that normal muscle will also show a decrease in amplitude providing the frequency of stimulation is high enough and the point at which this occurs and the extent to which it declines varies from subject to subject. Buchthal and his colleagues recently studied 23 patients and compared the electrical and mechanical responses with those of 30 normal subjects (Slomić *et al.*, 1968). They found that the best diagnostic procedures for myasthenia were the decrease in action potential amplitude and the absence of a staircase phenomenon when trains of stimuli were applied at 2–3/sec. for 90 sec. Twenty-two of 23 patients showed an abnormal mechanical response and 20 an abnormal electrical response. These results were positive in 7 out of 8 patients in whom the distal muscles were clinically uninvolved.

Pathology of muscle

Weigert (1901) was the first to describe lymphocytic infiltrations in the muscles of patients with myasthenia gravis and these were later given the name of lymphorrhage by Buzzard (1905). Dorothy Russell (1953) classified the types of lesion which may be seen in myasthenia gravis in her post-mortem study of the muscles of 8 patients. She found basically three types of lesion.

Type I. Acute coagulative necrosis of the muscle fibre, becoming initially swollen, with loss of nuclei and eosinophilia of the sarcoplasm. There is at first distortion, then loss of myofibrils and an intense inflammatory cellular reaction and ultimate phagocytosis of the fibre. These changes were found in 6 out of the 8 cases and were found mostly in the extraocular muscles, upper digestive tract, heart and diaphragm. In the 3 cases in which skeletal muscle was involved the changes were confined to trunk muscles.

Type II. Lymphorrhage formation. The earliest changes, affecting solitary muscle fibres, consisted of basophilia of the sarcoplasm and loss of cross striations. Later small numbers of lymphocytes gather about the disappearing fibre, until in the large lymphorrhage there is a mass of small lymphocytes and a few larger mononuclear cells with hardly any evidence of the residual basophilic fibre. These changes were found in all 8 cases, being present in the extra-ocular muscles of all 8 and in the limb muscles of 5.

Type III. A simple fibre atrophy of single muscle fibres or groups of fibres. There was no loss of cross-striations and no inflammatory cell infiltration. This type of change was seen in all of 8 patients and was most frequent in skeletal muscles.

Russell found that these muscle changes bore no relation to the presence or absence of a thymic tumour, but they did correlate quite well with the functional impairment demonstrated by the patients in life. The Type I and Type II changes seemed to be more important than the Type III.

More recently evidence has been forthcoming about these changes in two biopsy series (Fenichel, 1966; Engel and McFarlin, 1966). Type I changes were found in 7 to 32% of patients. The earliest Russell Type I change, that of "progressive atrophy" or "chronic necrosis" was found in 30% of Engel and McFarlin's series. The latter found the second stage of Russell Type II, that of lymphorrhages surrounding necrotic fibres, in 23% of their patients. Type III changes which were attributed to denervation and appeared as small, angulated groups of fibres on cross section were found in 30% of Fenichel's patients and in 63% of the series of Engel and McFarlin.

Genkins *et al.* (1961) in a post-mortem study of 31 cases of myasthenia gravis found muscle lesions in 24 (77%), and these were most pronounced in the 10 cases with thymoma.

Types of fibre atrophy

In the following paragraphs it should be noted that muscle fibre Types I and II refer to fibres which have been differentiated histochemically (Engel, 1965) and must not be confused with Russell's Type I, II and III changes. Engel and McFarlin (1966) found that in 50% of their patients, and in some with the above mentioned type of simple fibre atrophy, there was atrophy affecting Type II muscle fibres. Further work by Brooke and Engel (1969) on muscle biopsies of myasthenics has shown that both Type I and Type II fibres are reduced in size, but that the predominant change involves Type II fibres.

What do all these histological abnormalities mean? Dudgeon and Urquhart (1926) described atrophy of muscle fibres in association with lymphorrhages in 9 cases of Graves' disease, one of whom had also myasthenia gravis. Similar lymphorrhages in the muscles of thyrotoxic patients have been noted by several authors since then (Thorn and Eder, 1946; Hed, Kirstein and Lundmark, 1958; Whitfield and Hudson, 1961; Ramsay, 1964). Dorothy Russell (1953) was in some doubt about the meaning of these histological changes except that she concluded that they were intimately concerned in the muscular weakness and wasting. Simpson (1969) has suggested that the similarity of the changes in myasthenia gravis and in endocrine myopathy may be due to a common "auto-immune" mechanism. Brooke and Engel (1969), commenting on the reduction in size they found in Type II fibres, noted that this change was associated with many conditions in which the activity of muscles is limited; the Type I fibre atrophy was typical of denervation. Fenichel (1966) quoted evidence for the presence of denervation in myasthenia gravis and thought that those changes and those of an inflammatory myopathy were indicative of "auto-immune" disease.

Motor nerve endings

Using supravital staining techniques for the motor nerve endings it has been shown that there are two principal abnormalities in the innervation of myasthenic muscle (Coërs and Woolf, 1959; Woolf, 1969). These are:

1. The dystrophic type in which there is sprouting of subterminal axons with the formation of multiple end-plates, which are smaller than usual and distributed over a larger area of muscle fibres than normal. This type of change is particularly seen in muscles which have histological evidence of lymphorrhages, degeneration of fibres and fibre atrophy. The abnormalities in the end-plates may well be secondary to muscle abnormalities.

2. The dysplasic type in which there are relatively few end-plates. These are elongated and there is little evidence of axonal sprouting. The relationships of both these types of end-plate to the clinical state in myasthenia gravis remains obscure. It is however interesting that both marked sprouting of subterminal nerve fibres with the formation of several end-plates on single muscle fibres (Coërs and Woolf, 1959) and elongation of the end-plates (Woolf, 1969) have been found in thyrotoxic myopathy. Havard *et al.* (1963), in their study of the muscles of 35 patients with thyrotoxicosis, detected abnormalities in the terminal axon and end-plate in 77%. These consisted of clubbing of the motor end-plate and marked swellings of the terminal axons. The changes were sporadic rather than diffuse and correlated poorly with E.M.G. findings. Whether or not these changes are secondary to muscle fibre dysfunction itself or are produced directly by the effects of excess thyroid hormone is unknown.

It can be concluded that pathological changes are often seen in muscle biopsies from patients with myasthenia gravis and that the frequency increases when post-mortem tissue is examined, as one might expect. It is possible that the structural changes could be related to the "myopathic" stage of myasthenia gravis, in which there is muscle wasting and weakness which is not responsive to neostigmine (Simpson, 1968). How the changes come about is still a matter for speculation. Could they be caused by an autoimmune reaction to a common "myoid" antigen shared by both thymus and skeletal muscle (see p. 74) or are they caused by a direct toxic action of excessive "Thymin" (see p. 73) released from the thymus? (Goldstein and Mackay, 1969; Goldstein, 1968).

Pathology of the thymus

The normal thymus weighs 22 ± 13 gm (mean ± S.D.) at birth; it increases to 34 ± 15 gm at puberty and diminishes to 9 ± 8 gm in senescence (Goldstein and Mackay, 1969). It consists of a lattice-work of connected epithelial cells amongst which are situated many lymphocytes. The lymphocytes are most dense at the periphery of the gland and this area is called the cortex. The central part, which contains fewer lymphocytes is called the medulla. The medulla also contains specialized epithelial structures called Hassall's corpuscles and adjacent to these are large, round "myoid" cells which in early life have a morphology similar to that of striated muscle and at all ages react antigenically in the same way as skeletal muscles. The normal thymus contains few germinal centres or plasma cells. At birth the cortex occupies 60% of the thymus, but this diminishes to 30% at 70 years of age; there is also a decrease in the number of Hassall's corpuscles in the medulla from 12 per mm^2 at birth to 2 per mm^2 at the age of 70 (Goldstein and Mackay, 1967).

In myasthenia gravis

Castleman (1966) has summarized the thymic abnormalities found in myasthenia gravis. A thymoma is present in 10% of cases, 72% show an increased number of germinal centres in the medulla and only 18% appear entirely normal. Goldstein and Mackay (1969) have emphasized that the thymus of a patient with myasthenia gravis is usually not enlarged unless a thymoma is present. They performed quantitative studies on the thymuses of myasthenic patients who did not have a thymoma (Goldstein and Mackay, 1965). They found that there were no significant differences in thymic histology between the myasthenic patients and age matched controls apart from an increased number of medullary germinal centres and a greater density of plasma cells in the medulla (Goldstein, 1966a). On the basis of these results Goldstein (1966b) has suggested that the histological changes are due to chronic inflammation and he called the condition "thymitis".

In Thyrotoxicosis

An enlarged thymus in thyrotoxicosis has been recognized for about 50 years. Goldstein and Mackay (1969) quoted Hammar's work of 1929 in which he showed that the weight of the whole thymus and of the cortex and medulla separately were greater than normal at all ages studied (Fig. 2.5). Hammar (1929) also noted a parallel increase in Hassall's corpuscles in the thymic medulla. This increase in thymic size in thyrotoxicosis has been confirmed radiologically in patients (Irvine and Sumerling, 1965; Michie *et al.*, 1967).

Experimental animals have been shown to develop an increase in thymic size by the administration of thyroxine. This has been shown in rats by Houssay (1944) and in fowls by Hohn (1959) and Warner (1964). It has also been noted that the administration of antithyroid drugs to thyrotoxic patients caused a diminution in thymic size

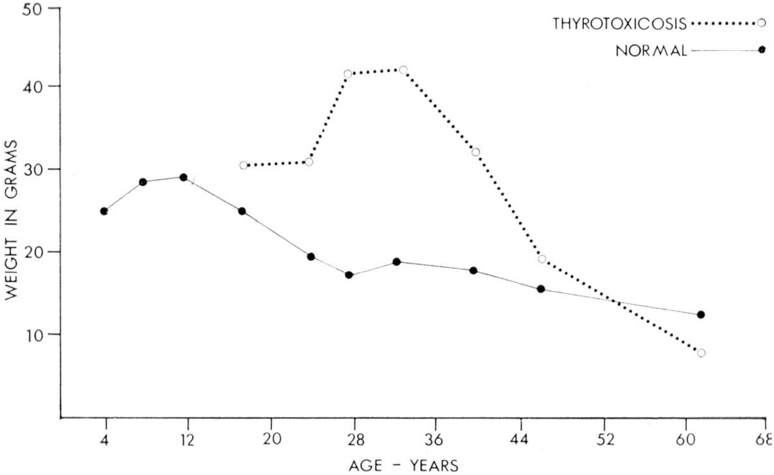

Figure 2.5. The weights of whole thymus plotted by age in "normal" subjects (cases of sudden death) and in thyrotoxic patients. (Modified from Mackay and Goldstein, 1966, data of Hammar, 1929).

(Michie *et al.*, 1967), suggesting that the enlarged thymus in thyrotoxicosis is a consequence of the increased amount of circulating thyroxine rather than an immunological factor such as Long Acting Thyroid Stimulator which is believed to be concerned in the aetiology of Graves' disease (Hetzel, 1968).

Gunn and his colleagues (1964) studied the histology of thymic biopsies performed during the course of operations for thyroid disease. They found that 32% of the patients with thyrotoxicosis had germinal centres in the thymic medulla compared with only 4% of patients with non-toxic goitre. There was no correlation with circulating thyroid autoantibodies but there was a relationship to the presence of germinal centres in the thyroid. This is further supportive evidence to suggest that the histological changes as well as the thymic size may be more related to elevated levels of thyroxine rather than to autoimmune factors.

Endocrine function of the thymus

The evidence for the production of a substance "thymin" by the thymus has been summarized by Goldstein and Mackay (1969). Repeated daily injections of thymin over a 10-day period into guinea pigs produced histological changes similar to the myopathic or myositic picture seen in myasthenia gravis. Moreover alterations in muscle tension in response to indirect stimulation were comparable to those in myasthenia gravis in that there was improvement with the addition of neostigmine and a very evident sensitivity to the blocking action of D-tubocurarine.

Thymin can be detected by the measurement of spontaneously occurring miniature end-plate potentials (m.e.p.p.) which are thought to be produced by the smallest amount (quantum) of neuromuscular transmitter (Fatt and Katz, 1952). Thymin reduces the amplitude of these m.e.p.p.s and a reduced amplitude is also found in myasthenia gravis (Hofmann and Stemmer, 1963) and in experimental auto-immune thymitis (Goldstein and Hofmann, 1968). Goldstein and Hofmann (1969) noted that neonatally thymectomized rats developed an increase in the m.e.p.p. amplitude, whereas rats who had had extra thymic tissue grafted showed a decrease in m.e.p.p. amplitude. There thus seems to be good evidence for the production of thymin by the thymus and for its action in producing neuromuscular block. The substance seems to be produced in excess in experimental auto-immune thymitis and Goldstein and Mackay (1969) postulate that this is the situation in myasthenia gravis itself.

Attention has been drawn earlier (p. 56) to the interrelationship between thyrotoxicosis and myasthenia gravis. In a majority of cases the later disease becomes worse as thyroid over-activity develops and improves as thyroid hormone levels are brought back to normal by treatment. Since thyroxine has been shown to cause thymic hyperplasia it might be speculated that this would cause an increase in the release of thymin by a gland which is already releasing excessive amounts because of the presence of auto-immune thymitis. The evidence that thymitis in myasthenia gravis is caused by auto-immune disease is based upon its similarity in many aspects to other auto-immune diseases. Myasthenia gravis is a disease commoner in women, occurring most frequently between the ages of 10 and 40 (Fig. 2.6), and like many other auto-immune diseases it is fluctuant in its course. Moreover, up to 51 % of patients with myasthenia gravis have been shown to have antibodies which react immunofluorescently with the A band of skeletal muscle (Downes, 1968). Namba *et al.* (1967) showed that if the patients' serum was made to react with preparations of their own muscle, then 9 out of 10 patients showed binding activity, the degree of which tended to be propor-

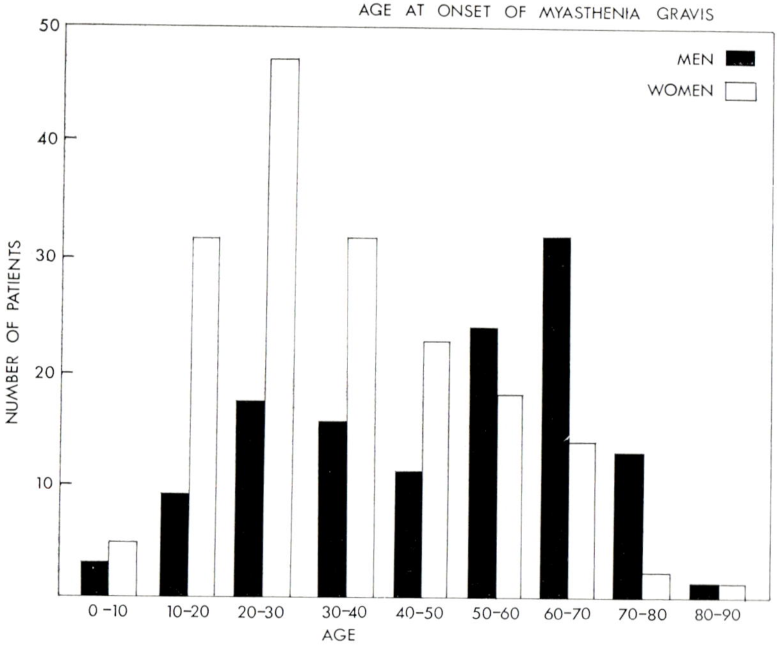

Figure 2.6. Age at onset, by decade, of myasthenia gravis in 295 patients. The commonest age of onset in women is in the third decade. (From Simpson *et al.*, 1966).

tional to the severity of the disease. Van der Geld and his colleagues (1964) showed that the antibody also reacted with certain cells in the thymus, now known to be myoid cells (Feltkamp-Vroom, 1966; Henry, 1966; Van de Velde, 1966). Furthermore, as Simpson pointed out in 1960 there is a significant coincidence of myasthenia gravis with other diseases of presumed auto-immune origin. This coincidence is most commonly found with Graves' disease, Hashimoto's thyroiditis and primary hypothyroidism (Simpson, 1968).

An additional factor suggesting that there is a link between myasthenia gravis and thyroid auto-immune disease is the presence of thyroid antibodies in about 24% of myasthenia patients (Table 2.7). The figures vary according to which antibody is being studied and by what method, but the prevalence of thyroid antibodies is significantly higher in the myasthenics than in control subjects (Downes, Greenwood and Wray, 1966; Vetters, 1967). It might be deduced from the data of Osserman, Tsairis and Weiner (1967) that, since 13·1% of their myasthenic patients had overt thyroid disease

TABLE 2.7

Thyroid antibodies in patients with myasthenia gravis

Authors	No. of patients	No. +ve	% +ve	Antibody and method
Van Der Geld *et al.*	111	36	32	Indirect immunofluorescence.
(1963)	81	9	11	Thyroglobulin haemagglutination.
Adner *et al.* (1964)	48	17	35	Thyroglobulin haemagglutination.
Sturgill *et al.* (1964)	41	3	7	Thyroglobulin haemagglutination.
Djanian *et al.* (1966)	70	12	17	Thyroglobulin haemagglutination.
Downes *et al.* (1966)	74	18	23	Thyroid cytoplasmic antibodies.
	74	10	14	Colloid antibodies.
	74	23	31	Thyroglobulin haemagglutination.
Simpson, J. A. (1966)	45	12	27	Not stated.
Wolf *et al.* (1966)	26	4	15	Thyroglobulin, method not stated.
Oosterhuis *et al.*	125		19	Colloid cytoplasm.
(1967)			14	Cytoplasm.
			28	One or both tests positive.
Vetters (1967)	89	20	22	Thyroid microsomal antibody.
Wright and Kerr (1967)	32	9	28	Thyroid cytoplasm, immunofluorescence.
	32	8	25	Thyroglobulin, tanned red cells.

and since these patients had a high prevalence of positive thyroid antibodies, this might account for the overall increase in positive thyroid antibodies in the general myasthenic population (Table 2.7). However, this cannot be the explanation, since, even when patients with overt thyroid disease were excluded, there were still significantly more patients than controls with positive antibodies (Table 2.8). Whether this implies that many myasthenic patients have subclinical thyroid disease remains to be seen. It is possible, for instance, that many patients with normal or borderline thyroid function tests may in fact be suffering from a mild degree of hypothyroidism as revealed by elevated TSH levels in blood (Hedley *et al.*, 1971).

TABLE 2.8

Thyroid antibodies in patients with myasthenia gravis (M.G.), myasthenia gravis plus thyroid disease, thyroid disease alone and in control subjects (derived from Osserman et al., *1967)*

Category	No. of patients	+ve immuno-fluorescence %	Significance	+ve haem-agglutination* %	Significance
M.G. alone	114	16·7	$p < 0{\cdot}05$	24·6	$p < 0{\cdot}001$
Controls	52	3·8		1·9	
M.G. + Thyroid disease	39	41	Not significant	46·2	Not significant
Thyroid disease alone	63	52·4		50·8	

* Positive between 1/25 and 1/2,500,000.

Thymoma and thyrotoxicosis

In 1960 James, Bowers and Ochsner reported the presence of an epithelial thymoma in a thyrotoxic patient. A thymolipoma was reported in another thyrotoxic in 1966 (Benton and Gerard, 1966). From these small numbers it would appear that the coincidence was fortuitous rather than related.

Thymectomy

Thymectomy is known to be of benefit in the management of myasthenia gravis (Simpson, 1958) but has been tried unsuccessfully in the past for the treatment of thyrotoxicosis (Goldstein and Mackay, 1969). However, in a recent report, thymectomy in a patient with concurrent myasthenia gravis and thyrotoxicosis ameliorated the former and cured the latter (De Groot *et al.*, 1967). The patient was a 20-year-old girl. Antithyroglobulin antibodies were present in a titre of 1/1,256,000. She had an enlarged thymus and electromyography revealed rapid fatigue of muscle strength. The thymus was irradiated with 3000 Rads, the thyroid being excluded from the field of radiation. Methimazole was given in a dosage of 10 mg q.i.d. As the patient became euthyroid the myasthenia became easier to control. After eight weeks of methimazole therapy thymectomy was carried out. Histologically the thymus showed lymphoid hyperplasia with germinal centres. Following the thymectomy no further antithyroid therapy was given, but the patient remained euthyroid and serum protein bound iodine estimations were normal. The antithyroglobulin titre fell to 1/612. Over a five-month period following operation there was improvement in the myasthenia gravis and a lowering of the dosage of pyridostigmine.

It is possible that the thyrotoxicosis went into spontaneous remission, though it would be unusual in such a short period as eight weeks. The dramatic drop in the antithyroglobulin titre at the same time as the remission of the thyrotoxicosis might suggest that the thymectomy had some effect on the thyrotoxicosis.

Myasthenia gravis, hypothyroidism and thyroiditis

In contrast to the well-recognized association of myasthenia gravis with thyrotoxicosis (see p. 53), the combination of hypothyroidism with myasthenia gravis is thought to be rare (Feinberg, Underdahl and Eaton, 1957; Namba and Grob, 1971), for myasthenia gravis has been reported as only occurring in 0·03% of 12,962 hypothyroid patients (Bartels and Kingsley, 1949). On the other hand, Sahay and his colleagues found hypothyroidism in nearly 2% of 260 patients with myasthenia gravis, and in their series noted that it was more common than thyrotoxicosis (Sahay, Blendis and Greene, 1965). These figures may be an underestimate, since they were derived from the records of patients attending during the previous 20 years and it was only in the last two years that tests for thyroid function were routinely performed in patients with myasthenia gravis. Rather similar figures were obtained by Storm-Mathisen in her series (1961) (Table 2.9). Sahay and his colleagues (1965) pointed out that hypo-

TABLE 2.9

The prevalence of hypothyroidism in patients with myasthenia gravis.

Authors	No. of patients with myasthenia gravis	No. of patients with hypo-thyroidism	Prevalence %
Storm-Mathisen (1961)	90	2	2·2
Sahay, Blendis and Greene (1965)	260	5	1·9
Simpson, Westerberg and Magee (1966)	295	16	5·8
Osserman *et al.* (1967)	801	46	5·7

thyroidism was quite likely to be unrecognized clinically in many cases. More systematic investigations into the thyroid status of myasthenic patients were carried out in two more recent series (Table 2.9), where it was revealed that nearly 6% had evidence of hypothyroidism (Simpson, Westerberg and Magee, 1966; Osserman, Tsairis and Weiner, 1967). Simpson (1968) in an examination of the thyroid function of 66 myasthenic patients found evidence of sub-clinical hypothyroidism in 4 (6%). It seems from these figures that hypothyroidism, latent or apparent, is just as common in myasthenic patients as is thyrotoxicosis (see Table 2.2, p. 54).

Without systematic thyroid antibody and biopsy studies it is difficult to know how many of the hypothyroid patients had Hashimoto's disease. At least 11 myasthenia gravis patients have been described with apparent Hashimoto's disease (Boshes and Mier, 1961; Greenberg, 1964; Daly and Jackson, 1964; Simpson, 1964, 1966; Singer and Sahay, 1966; Osserman, Tsairis and Weiner, 1967; Dunston, 1969). This small number of reported cases gives the impression that thyroiditis is rare in myasthenia gravis, yet Simpson

(1968) found clinically apparent Hashimoto's disease in 2 out of 66 patients (3%).

Pathologically 17% of the thyroid glands removed from myasthenic patients at autopsy have the histological changes of Hashimoto's thyroiditis according to Ringertz (1951). In another autopsy series (Becker *et al.*, 1964) 19% of myasthenic patients had evidence of Hashimoto's disease compared to 0·9% of 15,672 controls. Wolf *et al.* (1966) found changes of thyroiditis in 12% of their autopsy series, though none had had clinical evidence of thyroiditis. This pathological evidence, coupled with the finding of positive immunofluorescent tests and haemagglutination tests for thyroid antibodies in 16·7% and 24·6% respectively of patients with myasthenia gravis, compared with 3·8% and 1·9% of controls (Table 2.8) would make it seem likely that about 16% of myasthenic patients have thyroiditis, though in the majority it does not produce any clinical manifestations.

The thymus in myasthenic patients with Hashimoto's thyroiditis or myxoedema

Simpson (1968), in his study of 518 patients with myasthenia gravis found evidence of a thymoma in one out of 6 patients with Hashimoto's disease and in one out of 2 patients with hypothyroidism. This prevalence is much higher than he found in thyrotoxic patients (2 out of 37).

Effect of hypothyroidism on myasthenia

There is no specific temporal relationship between the onset of hypothyroidism and myasthenia gravis. In a review of 8 patients with the two diseases Bronsky, Meltzer and Waldstein (1967) found that, of the 2 men and 6 women studied, the myasthenia gravis preceded the hypothyroidism in 3 patients, occurred simultaneously in 2 and followed it in 3. There appeared to be no relationship between the severity of the hypothyroidism and myasthenia gravis in any of the cases and they noted that the treatment of the myasthenia gravis had no effect on the hypothyroidism. The converse was however also true; that replacement therapy for the hypothyroidism did not seem to improve the myasthenia gravis. This is rather strange, for in patients with myasthenia gravis and thyrotoxicosis who have been over-treated, there does appear to be a relationship. Monro (1963) described a female patient aged 26 who had thyrotoxicosis and myasthenia gravis. Too much treatment with carbimazole lowered her serum protein-bound iodine to 1·7 µg % and her myasthenia

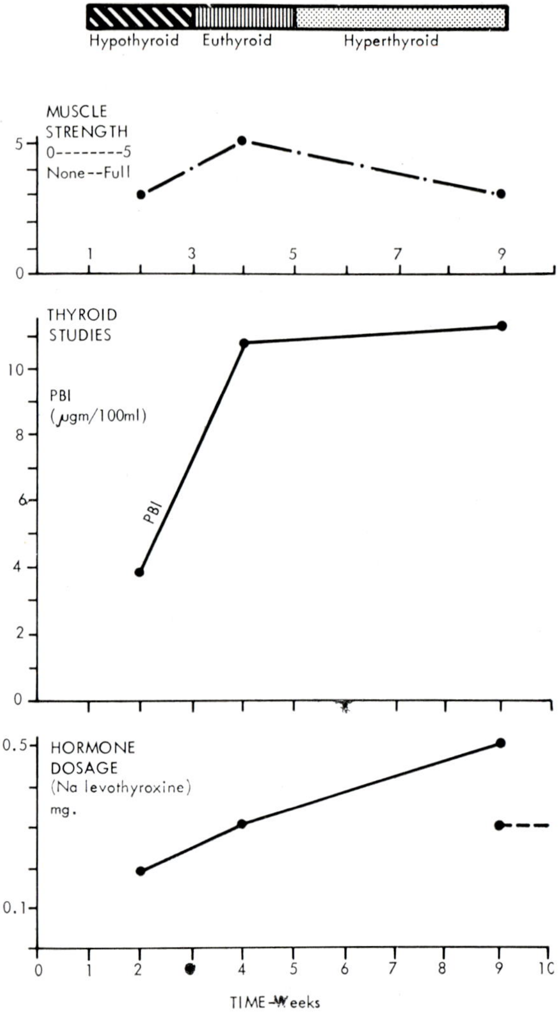

Figure 2.7. The effect of hypothyroidism, euthyroidism and hypothyroidism on the muscle strength of a patient with myasthenia gravis and thyrotoxicosis who became hypothyroid following radioactive iodine treatment. (Modified from Gaelen and Levitan, 1968).

gravis became much worse. When the P.B.I. had risen to 3·9 μg % the myasthenia improved. A further example is Gaelen and Levitan's (1968) patient, a 41-year-old woman, who presented with ptosis and blurring of vision. Investigations suggested that she had thyrotoxicosis and she was given 15·2 mC of radioactive iodine as therapy. She also received 180 mg of pyridostigmine daily. Within a month she developed evidence of hypothyroidism and her myasthenia gravis became worse in that she had weakness of extension and flexion of her fingers and a diminution of power in her shoulder girdle muscles. There was a great improvement in these symptoms when she was started on L-Thyroxine replacement, but a further worsening as the patient was made toxic on 0·5 mg per day. When the dose was reduced to 0·3 mg the muscle status returned to the same as that when she was previously euthyroid (see Fig. 2.7). Their findings confirmed those of Drachman (1962) who found that any deviation from the euthyroid state, either hyper or hypo, caused a worsening of myasthenia gravis.

Association of myasthenia gravis with other thyroid disease

Osserman and his colleagues (1967) found that 17 out of 801 patients with myasthenia gravis had a non-toxic goitre, a prevalence of 2·1%. Simpson (1968) noted that 7% of his 518 patients had non-toxic goitres and that 10 patients had had a goitre some time in the past. Simpson (1968) considered this to be a true association, but this must be interpreted with caution since there is a variable

TABLE 2.10

The prevalence of non-toxic goitre in autopsies of patients with myasthenia gravis

Authors	No. of myasthenic patients	No. with non-toxic goitre	%
Ringertz (1951)	18	1	5·5
Rowland *et al.* (1956)	26	4	15
Genkins *et al.* (1961)	31	4	12·5

prevalence of goitre in different parts of the world. Simpson's patients presumably came from London, Edinburgh and Glasgow, not notably goitrous areas. They are comparable with the North East of England when the prevalence of goitre in the "normal" population is 9% of women and 1% of men (Hall, Anderson and

Smart, 1969). These figures are fairly close to those for non-toxic goitre found in post-mortem series of myasthenic patients (Table 2.10), and suggest that the relationship between non-toxic goitre and myasthenia gravis is no higher than would be expected in the general population. However, the finding by Kotylarov, Gilin and Morgunova (1969) of iodine deficiency goitre with euthyroidism in 56 out of 172 Soviet patients with myasthenia gravis cannot be ignored and obviously more work is needed to clarify the association.

Hereditary factors

Hyperthyroidism is thought in some way to be genetically transmitted (Bartels, 1941; Martin and Fisher, 1945). Strong evidence for this was provided by Verschuer (1959) who found the concordant occurrence of hyperthyroidism in 47% of 49 pairs of monozygotic twins, but in only 3% of 64 pairs of dizygotic twins. Namba and Grob (1971) noted that there was also some tendency for myasthenia gravis to run in families, in that 3% of all myasthenic patients have a positive family history.

Among patients suffering from both myasthenia gravis and overt thyroid disease, there is a remarkably high family prevalence of the two conditions. Out of 20 patients with myasthenia gravis and hyperthyroidism, Rowland, Aranow and Hoefer (1966) found that two of their patients had siblings who were also affected by thyrotoxicosis. In one family three siblings had had thyrotoxicosis and two of them also had myasthenia gravis. A strong association between myasthenia gravis and thyrotoxicosis was also noted by Namba and Grob (1971). They described one sister who developed myasthenia gravis shortly after becoming hypothyroid as a result of sub-total thyroidectomy. The other got myasthenia gravis and thyrotoxicosis at the same time. They had a brother with thyrotoxicosis alone. Macrae (1954) described a myasthenic child whose mother had hyperthyroidism. Greenberg (1964) reported two sisters with thyrotoxicosis and myasthenia gravis, one of whom became hypothyroid after radioactive iodine therapy; the other developed Hashimoto's disease with hypothyroidism six years after the onset of thyrotoxicosis. Simpson (1968) had one male patient with myasthenia whose twin sister had a goitre. Namba and Grob (1971) calculated from their own cases and from those published in the literature that the prevalence of hyperthyroidism in familial myasthenia gravis is 3%. Namba and Grob did not consider that thyroid disorder was more commonly associated with familial myasthenia than with the non-familial disease.

Simpson (1960) was really the first to note the general association of thyroid disease with myasthenia gravis. He found a family history of toxic or non-toxic goitre or of hypothyroidism in 20 of 440 cases of myasthenia gravis and commented that the exact prevalence was uncertain since he had only systematically questioned patients on this subject since 1953. The supposition is that the association may be even more frequent than he found. From Simpson's observations it appears that the relative with thyroid disease was usually a sister or a female on either the maternal or paternal side of the family. Oosterhuis (1964) recorded 10 instances of thyroid disorder among the close relatives (parents, children, sisters and brothers) of 110 myasthenic patients.

It seems clear from the evidence put forward in previous sections of this chapter that myasthenia gravis does not cause thyroid disease or vice versa, but that they both occur in patients who have a predilection to develop the two. As has been shown on p. 53, myasthenic patients are more likely to develop thyrotoxicosis than the general population and the converse is also true. The same probably applies to hypothyroidism and Hashimoto's disease. Even in myasthenic patients with no clinical evidence of thyroid disease positive haemagglutination tests for thyroglobulin antibody were found in nearly 25% compared with only 2% of controls (Osserman, Tsairis and Weiner, 1967). Graves' disease, Hashimoto's disease and even idiopathic hypothyroidism are associated with a high incidence of thyroid auto-antibodies (Roitt and Doniach, 1960) and are now generally accepted as being auto-immune in origin. Other auto-immune diseases such as rheumatoid arthritis (Simpson, 1960; White and Marshall, 1962; Van der Geld *et al.*, 1963), pernicious anaemia (Reaves, 1965; Simpson, 1966; Durston, 1969), Sjögren's disease (Simpson, 1968) and systemic lupus erythrematosus (Wolf *et al.*, 1966; Simpson, 1966) have all been reported in patients with myasthenia gravis, just as they have been in patients with Graves' disease.

The link, therefore, between different diseases of auto-immune origin is strong and there appears to be some hereditary basis to it, though the exact genetics are uncertain. Simpson (1960) originally suggested that a gene may have a variable expression, sometimes producing thyroid disease, sometimes myasthenia gravis, occasionally both or it could act on immunological responses via the thymus. Burnet (1959) has put forward the theory that the auto-immune diseases are due to the emergence, in some genetically predisposed persons, of "forbidden clones", so that the immune mechanisms of the body are unable to recognize "self". The result is antibody formation. So far there is little conclusive evidence as to whether auto-antibodies are the cause or the result of tissue damage, except that it is known that the thyroid overactivity of Graves' disease is something to do with a stimulating antibody called Long Acting Thyroid Stimulator (Hetzel, 1968) and that myasthenia gravis has been produced in animals by the administration of serum containing antibody to striped muscle (Goldstein and Mackay, 1969).

The site of action of thyroid hormone in myasthenia gravis

Namba and Grob (1971) have recently analysed the inter-relationships of 153 patients with myasthenia gravis and thyrotoxicosis reported in the literature. Effective treatment for the thyrotoxicosis, or a spontaneous remission of the disease, improved the myasthenia in 62% of patients, 5 of whom had also had thymectomy carried out. In 38% of the myasthenics the disease became worse with the control of the thyrotoxicosis. Although Grob (1958) found that the administration of thyroid hormone to 7

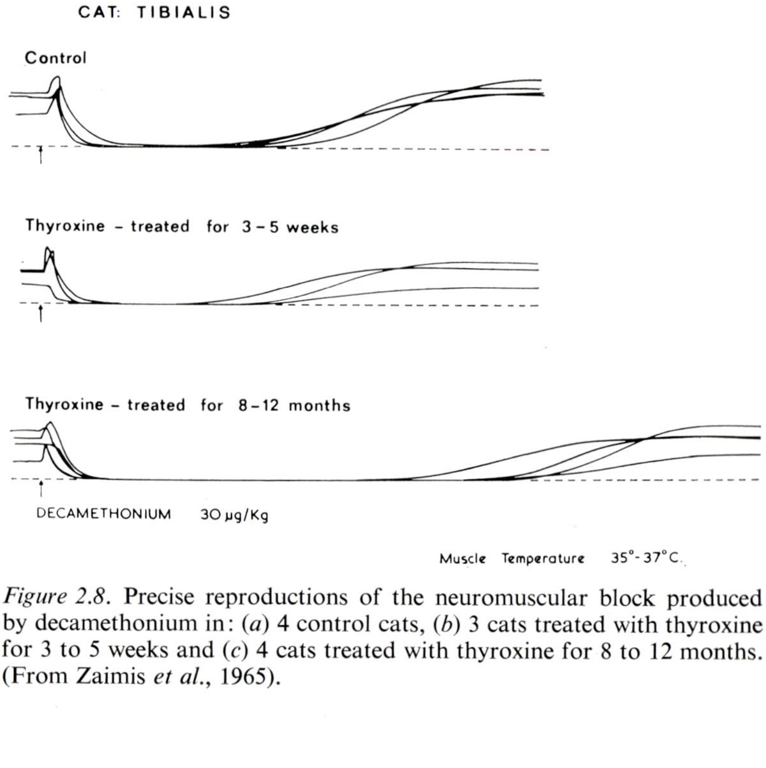

Figure 2.8. Precise reproductions of the neuromuscular block produced by decamethonium in: (*a*) 4 control cats, (*b*) 3 cats treated with thyroxine for 3 to 5 weeks and (*c*) 4 cats treated with thyroxine for 8 to 12 months. (From Zaimis *et al.*, 1965).

euthyroid patients made no difference to the myasthenia in 6, others have found that both an excess and a deficiency of thyroxine have a deleterious effect on the myasthenia (Engel, 1961; Drachman, 1962; Monro, 1963; Gaelen and Levitan, 1968). Is this due to the effects of an excess or a deficiency of thyroid hormone on end-plate function or is it merely that the effects of thyrotoxic or hypothyroid myopathy are grafted on to those of myasthenia gravis?

Zaimis and her colleagues who studied neuromuscular function in cats before and after treatment with thyroxine found that after

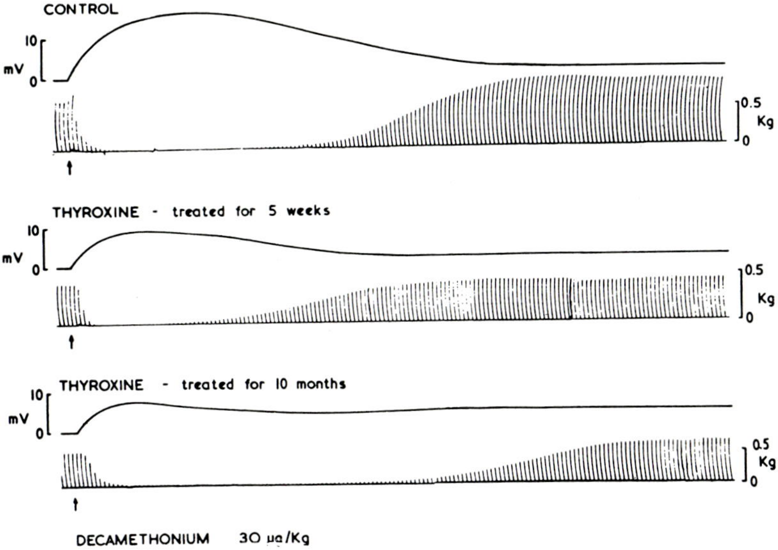

Figure 2.9. Tibialis anterior muscle. Records of depolarisation of the end-plate region (measured with an external electrode) and of twitch tension in response to decamethonium in control and thyroxine-treated cats. (From Zaimis *et al.*, 1965).

after four to six weeks of thyroxine treatment all animals showed a myopathic pattern, with shortening of motor unit action potentials (Zaimis *et al.*, 1965). The maximum twitch tension was smaller in the thyroxine-treated animals, but the time course of the twitch was not significantly different from that of the control animals. In control and treated animals the sensitivity of the muscle to anticholinesterase and depolarizing drugs was unchanged or increased. However, in the thyroxine-treated cats there was a decrease in the rate of recovery from neuromuscular block induced by decamethonium (Fig. 2.8). This effect increased the longer the treatment was continued. The reduced recovery from neuromuscular block was accompanied by a slowing of the rate of the repolarization phase (Fig. 2.9). Zaimis and her colleagues concluded that the functional defect produced by thyroxine appeared to be on the muscle fibre and not at the neuromuscular junction.

Not a lot of information is available about the effect in thyrotoxics of alterations in the concentrations of calcium and magnesium on motor end-plate function. The work of Del Castillo and Katz (1954a, b) and of Jenkinson (1957) suggests that acetylcholine release, as a result of nerve impulses, is under some degree of control by a calcium-containing compound. More acetylcholine may be released if the concentration of calcium is raised or that of magnesium is lowered. It is thought that calcium and magnesium may compete for the same receptor site or for a carrier molecule.

Kornfeld, Somlyo and Osserman (1969) have studied the effect of calcium gluconate infusion on the muscle strength of 10 patients with myasthenia gravis and of 10 controls. The calcium made no difference to the controls but improved muscle strength in 6 out of the 10 myasthenics. The effect appeared within three to six minutes and lasted for between 15 and 45 minutes. The improvement varied from 20 to 59% above the baseline measurements of hand ergograms and the size of palpebral fissures and affected both skeletal and bulbar musculature. One patient with both myasthenia gravis and thyrotoxicosis has been studied by George and Haan (1962). One gram of intravenous calcium gluconate, half the dose used by Kornfeld, Somlyo and Osserman (1969), produced an immediate but transient increase in strength. The patient was then put on magnesium sulphate by mouth, but after just over two days it had to be stopped because she became so weak. She was given calcium lactate 2·4 g daily by mouth and within five days she was as strong as before the administration of magnesium. The calcium treatment was continued and a progressive increase in muscle strength persisted. Kornfeld, Somlyo and Osserman (1969) suggested that the action of the calcium was to increase the number of quanta released by single nerve impulses. Alterations in the calcium to magnesium ratio change the quantal output initiated by each impulse.

Another way in which thyrotoxicosis may be associated with a worsening of myasthenia gravis is the finding of abnormal end plates in 77% of patients with uncomplicated thyrotoxicosis (Havard *et al.*, 1963). These structural abnormalities may conceivably increase the defect in neuromuscular transmission which is characteristic of myasthenia gravis. The morphological changes are reversible after the treatment of thyrotoxicosis (Devic, 1947) and, since a majority of myasthenics improve at this time, this is supportive evidence for a causal relationship.

Massari, Guardamagna and Bertolini (1958) found that the true muscle cholinesterase was increased in rats made hyperthyroid with thyroid hormone. They discovered that the reverse was true in hypothyroidism. It might be thought that this could partly explain the worsening of myasthenia gravis in the majority of patients who develop concomitant thyrotoxicosis (Boshes and Mier, 1961). However it is difficult to reconcile with the inference of Tabachnick and his colleagues that hyperthyroidism causes an increase in the production of acetylcholine and that the muscle weakness of hyperthyroidism may be in part due to the depolarizing action of excess acetylcholine (Tabachnick *et al.*, 1958). The latter authors found that hyperthyroid animals were significantly more sensitive to decamethonium and neostigmine when compared to saline treated animals. Although antagonism to d-tubocurarine would have been expected if acetylcholine concentrations were increased in the motor end-plates, in fact none was found. McCorkle (1952) also found no increased sensitivity to d-tubocurarine in thyrotoxic patients. Tabachnick *et al.* (1958) commented that a mechanism by which there was sensitivity to decamethonium and a normal response to d-tubocurarine remained unknown.

Conclusions

There is no evidence that thyroid disease causes myasthenia gravis. It is more likely that they occur together in the same individual because that individual is genetically predisposed to auto-immune disease. However, in the majority of patients the development of either hyper- or hypothyroidism will tend to make the myasthenia gravis more severe. The mechanisms by which this happens could be those of altered motor end-plate morphology, changes in the ratio of calcium to magnesium, or alterations in the production of acetylcholine and cholinesterase; though it is much more likely that the worsening of the myasthenia is due to the additional burden of a hyper- or hypothyroid myopathy, which is present in a large number of patients with these diseases.

REFERENCES

Adner, M. M., Sherman, J. D., Isé, C., Schwab, R. S. and Dameshek, W. (1964). An immunologic survey of forty-eight patients with Myasthenia Gravis. *New Engl. J. Med.*, **271,** 1327.

Anderson, J. R., Gray, K. G., Middleton, D. G. and Young, J. A. (1964). Auto-immunity and thyrotoxicosis. *Brit. med. J.*, **2,** 1630.

Bartels, E. D. (1941). "Heredity in Graves' Disease". Munksgaard, Copenhagen.

Bartels, E. C. and Kingsley, J. W. Jr. (1949). Hyperthyroidism associated with myasthenia gravis. *Lahey Clin. Found. Bull.*, **6,** 101.

Becker, K. L., Titus, J. L., McConahey, W. M. and Woolner, L. B. (1964). Morphologic evidence of thyroiditis in myasthenia gravis. *J. Amer. med. Ass.*, **187,** 994.

Benton, C. and Gerard, P. (1966). Thymolipoma in a patient with Graves' disease. Case report and review of the literature. *J. thorac. cardiov. Surg.*, **51,** 428.

Boshes, B. and Mier, M. (1961). Myasthenic states and disturbances of thyroid metabolism. In "Myasthenia Gravis". Second International Symposium Proceedings. p. 467. Charles C. Thomas, Springfield, Illinois.

Brain, Lord and Walton, J. N. (1969). In "Brain's Diseases of the Nervous System", p. 864. Oxford University Press, London.

Bronsky, D., Meltzer, J. L. and Waldstein, S. S. (1967). Idiopathic juvenile myxedema and myasthenia gravis. A case with circulating thyroid and skeletal muscle antibodies. *Amer. J. Med.*, **43,** 956.

Brooke, M. H. and Engel, W. K. (1969). The histographic analysis of human muscle biopsies with regard to fiber types. 3. Myotonias, myasthenia gravis and hypokalemic periodic paralysis. *Neurology (Minneap.)*, **19,** 469.

Buchthal, F. (1970). Electrophysiological abnormalities in metabolic myopathies and neuropathies. *Acta neurol. scand.*, **46,** Supp. 43, 129.

Burnet, F. M. (1959). "The Clonal Selection Theory of Acquired Immunity." University Press, Cambridge.

Buzzard, E. F. (1905). The clinical history and post-mortem examination of five cases of myasthenia gravis. *Brain*, **28,** 438.

Castleman, B. (1966). The pathology of the thymus gland in myasthenia gravis. *Ann. N.Y. Acad. Sci.*, **135,** 496,

Churchill-Davidson, H. C. and Richardson, A. T. (1952). The action of decamethonium iodide (C. 10) in myasthenia gravis. *J. Neurol. Neurosurg. Psychiat.*, **15,** 129.

Coërs, C. and Woolf, A. L. (1959). "The Innervation of Muscle", pp. 100–18. Blackwell, Oxford.

Cohen, B. (1946). Thyrotoxicosis and myasthenia gravis: report of a case. *S. Afr. med. J.*, **20,** 408.

Daly, J. J. and Jackson, E. (1964). Case of Hashimoto's Disease with myasthenia gravis. *Brit. med. J.*, *i*, 748.

De Groot, L. J., Perlo, V., Gephart, T. and Schwab, R. (1967). Remission of myasthenia and thyrotoxicosis after thymectomy. *Ann. intern. Med.*, **67,** 1042.

Del Castillo, J. and Katz, B. (1954a). The effect of magnesium on the activity of motor nerve endings. *J. Physiol.*, **124,** 553.

Del Castillo, J. and Katz, B. (1954b). Changes in end-plate activity produced by presynaptic polarization. *J. Physiol.*, **124,** 586.

Devic, A., Froment, R., Guinet, P. and Devic, M. (1947). Les dystrophies musculaires hyperthyroïdiennes. À propos de 14 observations personnelles de myopathie basedowenne. *J. Méd. Lyon*, **28,** 155.

Djanian, A. Y., Witebsky, E. and Beutner, E. H. (1966). Formalinized tanned cell haemagglutination test for demonstration of autoantibodies in myasthenia gravis. *Proc. Soc. exp. Biol.*, **123,** 80.

Downes, J. M. (1968). Muscle auto-antibodies in myasthenia gravis. In "Research in muscular dystrophy". Proceedings IVth Symposium, January 1968. Editors: Members of the Research Committee of the Muscular Dystrophy Group. Pitman Medical Publishing Co. Ltd., London.

Downes, J. M., Greenwood B. M. and Wray, S. H. (1966). Autoimmune aspects of myasthenia gravis. *Quart. J. Med.*, **35,** 85.

Drachman, D. B. (1962). Myasthenia gravis and the thyroid gland. *New Eng. J. Med.*, **266,** 330.

Dudgeon, L. S. and Urquhart, A. L. (1926). Lymphorrhages in the muscles in exophthalmic goitre. *Brain*, **49,** 182.

Durston, J. H. J. (1969). Myasthenia gravis, Hashimoto's disease and pernicious anaemia. *Postgrad. med. J.*, **45,** 290.

Engel, A. G. (1961). Thyroid function and myasthenia gravis. *Arch. Neurol.*, **4,** 663.

Engel, W. K. (1965). "Histochemistry of neuromuscular disease. Significance of muscle fibre types". In Proceedings of the 8th Congress of Neurology, Vienna, Volume 2, Neuromuscular Diseases, p.67. Wiener Medizinische Akademie, Vienna.

Engel, W. K. and McFarlin, D. E. (1966). In discussion of Fenichel, G. M., "Muscle Lesions in Myasthenia Gravis". *Ann. N.Y. Acad. Sci.*, **135,** 68.

Fatt, P. and Katz, B. (1952). Spontaneous sub-threshold activity at motor nerve endings. *J. Physiol.*, **117,** 109.

Faurschou (1970), quoted by Buchthal (1970).

Feinberg, W. D., Underdahl, L. O. and Eaton, L. M. (1957). Myasthenia gravis and myxedema. *Proc. Mayo Clin.*, **32,** 299.

Feltkamp-Vroom, T. (1966). Myoid cells in human thymus. *Lancet*, *i*, 1320.

Fenichel, G. M. (1966). Muscle lesions in myasthenia gravis. *Ann. N.Y. Acad. Sci.*, **135,** 60.

Flynn, R. (1944). Graves' disease with disassociation of thyrotoxicosis and ophthalmopathy associated with myasthenia gravis. *Med. J. Aust.*, *i*, 344.

Gaelen, L. H. and Levitan, S. (1968). Myasthenia gravis and thyroid function. *Arch. Neurol.*, **18,** 107.

Garland, H. and Clark, A. N. G. (1956). Myasthenia gravis, a personal study of 60 cases. *Brit. med. J.*, *i*, 1259.

Genkins, G., Mendelow, H., Sobel, H. J. and Osserman, K. E. (1961). Myasthenia gravis: analysis of thirty-one consecutive post-mortem examinations. In "Myasthenia Gravis". Proceedings 2nd International Symposium, Los Angeles, 1959. Edited by H. R. Viets, p. 519. C. C. Thomas, Springfield, Illinois.

George, W. K. and Haan, C. L. (1962). Calcium and magnesium administration in myasthenia gravis. *Lancet*, *ii*, 561.

Glaser, G. H. (1966). Crisis, precrisis and drug resistance in myasthenia gravis. *Ann. N.Y. Acad. Sci.*, **135,** 335.

Goldstein, G. (1966a). Plasma cells in the human thymus. *Aust. J. exp. Biol. med. Sci.*, **44,** 695.

Goldstein, G. (1966b). Thymitis and myasthenia gravis. *Lancet*, *ii*, 1164.

Goldstein, G. (1968). The thymus and neuromuscular function. A substance in thymus which causes myositis and myasthenic neuromuscular block in guinea pigs. *Lancet*, *ii*, 119.

Goldstein, G. and Hofman, W. W. (1968). Electrophysiological changes similar to those of myasthenia gravis in rats with experimental autoimmune thymitis. *J. Neurol. Neurosurg. Psychiat.*, **31,** 453.

Goldstein, G. and Hofman, W. W. (1969). Endocrine function of the thymus affecting neuromuscular transmission. *Clin. exp. Immunol.*, **4,** 181.

Goldstein, G. and Mackay, I. R. (1965). Contrasting abnormalities in the thymus in systemic lupus erythematosus and myasthenia gravis: a quantitative histological study. *Aust. J. exp. Biol. med. Sci.*, **43,** 381.

Goldstein, G. and Mackay, I. R. (1967). The thymus in systemic lupus erythematosus. A quantitative histopathological analysis and comparison with stress involution. *Brit. med. J.*, *ii*, 475.

Goldstein, G. and Mackay, I. R. (1969). "The human thymus." Heinemann, London.

Greenberg, J. (1964). Myasthenia gravis and hyperthyroidism in two sisters. *Arch. Neurol.*, **11,** 219.

Greene, R. (1949). Thyrotoxicosis, exophthalmic ophthalmoplegia, myasthenia gravis and vitiligo. *Proc. roy. Soc. Med.*, **42,** 263.

Grob, D. (1958). Myasthenia gravis. Current status of pathogenesis, clinical manifestations and management. *J. chron. Dis.*, **8,** 536.

Grob, D. and Harvey, A. McG. (1953). Abnormalities in neuromuscular transmission, with special reference to myasthenia gravis. *Amer. J. Med.*, **15,** 695.

Gunn, A., Michie, W. and Irvine, W. J. (1964). The thymus in thyroid disease. *Lancet*, *ii*, 776.

Hall, R., Anderson, J. and Smart, G. A. (1969). "Fundamentals of Clinical Endocrinology," p. 76. Pitman Medical, London.

Hammar (1929), quoted by Goldstein and Mackay (1969).

Hatch, H. A. (1952). Myasthenia gravis: report of a case with exophthalmos, without hyperthyroidism, relieved by neostigmine. *New Eng. J. Med.*, **246,** 856.

Havard, C. W. H., Campbell, E. D. R., Ross, H. B. and Spence, A. W. (1963). Electromyographic and histological findings in the muscles of patients with thyrotoxicosis. *Quart. J. Med.*, **32,** 145.

Hed, R., Kirstein, L. and Lundmark, C. (1958). Thyrotoxic myopathy. *J. Neurol. Neurosurg. Psychiat.*, **21,** 270.

Hedley, A. J., Hall, R., Amos, J., Michie, W. and Crooks, J. (1971). Serum thyrotropin levels after subtotal thyroidectomy for Graves' Disease. *Lancet*, *i*, 455.

Henry, K. (1966). Mucin secretion and striated muscle in the human thymus. *Lancet*, *i*, 183.

Hetzel, B. S. (1968). The aetiology and pathogenesis of hyperthyroidism. *Postgrad. med. J.*, **44,** 363.

Hofmann, W. W. and Stemmer, E. A. (1963). Subthreshold activity at normal and myasthenic end-plates. *Neurology* (*Minneap.*), **13,** 227.

Höhn, E. O. (1959). Actions of certain hormones on the thymus of the domestic hen. *J. Endocrinol.*, **19,** 282.

Houssay (1944). Unpublished work quoted by Rapela (1944).

Irvine, W. J. and Sumerling, M. D. (1965). Radiological assessment of the thymus in thyroid and other diseases. *Lancet*, *i*, 996.

Iversen, K. (1948). "Temporary Rise in the Frequency of Thyrotoxicosis in Denmark 1941–45." Rosenkilde and Bagger, Copenhagen.

James, T. N., Bowers, C. Y. and Ochsner, A. (1960). Some cardiac problems presented by a thymoma. *Dis. Chest*, **38,** 193.

Jenkinson, D. H. (1957). The nature of the antagonism between calcium and magnesium ions at the neuromuscular junction. *J. Physiol.*, **138,** 434.

Joasoo, A., Murray, I. P. C. and Steinbeck, A. W. (1970). Involvement of bulbar muscles in thyrotoxic myopathy. *Aust. Ann. Med.*, **19,** 338.

Kissel, P., Hartemann, P. and Duc, M. (1965). "Les Syndromes Myo-thyroïdiens." Masson, Paris.

Kissel, P., Schmitt, J., Duc, M. and Duc, M. L. (1970). Myasthenia and thyrotoxicosis. In "Proceedings of an International Congress on Muscle Diseases, Milan, 1969". Edited by J. N. Walton, N. Canal and G. Scarlato, p. 464. Excerpta Medica, Amsterdam.

Kornfeld, P., Somlyo, A. and Osserman, K. E. (1969). Role of calcium in myasthenia gravis. *Arch. Neurol.* (*Chic.*), **21,** 466.

Kotlyarov, E. V., Gilin, M. M. and Morgunova, T. I. (1969). Study of the thyroid profile in patients suffering from myasthenia. (*Russ.*). *Probl. Endokr.*, **15,** No. 6, 23.

Kowallis, G. F., Haines, S. F. and Pemberton, J. J. (1942). Goiter with associated myasthenia gravis: report of three cases of exophthalmic goiter and one case of adenomatous goiter with hyperthyroidism. *Arch. intern. Med.*, **69,** 41.

Lahey, F. H. (1926). Quadriceps test for the myasthenia of thyroidism. *J. Amer. med. Ass.*, **87,** 754.

Logan, W. P. D. and Cushion, A. A. (1958). "Studies on Medical and Population Subjects" (No. 14). Morbidity Statistics from General Practice. Vol. I. (General). Her Majesty's Stationery Office, London.

McCorkle, J. K. (1952). Myasthenia gravis and exophthalmic goitre. Thesis, University of Minnesota Graduate School, Minneapolis.

McEachern, D. and Parnell, J. L. (1948). The relationship of hyperthyroidism to myasthenia gravis. *J. clin. Endocr.*, **8,** 842.

McEachern, D. and Ross, W. D. (1942). Chronic thyrotoxic myopathy: a report of three cases with a review of previously reported cases. *Brain*, **65,** 181.

Maclean, B. and Wilson, J. A. C. (1954). See-saw relationship between hyperthyroidism and myasthenia gravis. *Lancet*, *i*, 950.

Macrae, D. (1954). Myasthenia gravis in early childhood. *Pediatrics*, **13,** 511.

Martin, L. and Fisher, R. A. (1945). The hereditary and familial aspects of exophthalmic goitre and nodular goitre. *Quart. J. Med.*, **14,** 207.

Massari, N., Guardamagna, C. and Bertolini, A. M. (1958). L'ormone tiroideo e la vera colinesterasi del tessuto muscolare e del tessuto cerebrale. *Acta vitamin.* (*Milano*), **12,** 13.

Means, J. H., De Groot, L. J. and Stanbury, J. B. (1963). In "The Thyroid and its Diseases", p. 170. McGraw-Hill, New York.

Melville, I. D. (1959). Chronic thyrotoxic myopathy. *Scot. med. J.*, **4,** 318.

Michie, W., Beck, J. S., Mahaffy, R. G., Honein, E. F. and Fowler, G. B. (1967). Quantitative radiological and histological studies of the thymus in thyroid disease. *Lancet*, *i*, 691.

Millikan, C. H. and Haines, S. F. (1953). The thyroid gland in relation to neuromuscular disease. *Arch. intern. Med.*, **92,** 5.

Monro, P. (1963). Treatment of myasthenia gravis. *Lancet*, *i*, 108.

Nakao, K., Sekihara, H., Uchimura, H. *et al.* (1967). A case of myasthenia gravis complicated by Hashimoto's thyroiditis and atrophic gastritis. (*Jap*). *Naika.*, **20,** 973.

Namba, T., Brunner, N. G., Brown, S. B., Muguruma, M. and Grob, D. (1971). Familial myasthenia gravis. Report of 27 patients in 12 families and review of 164 patients in 73 families. *Arch. Neurol.* (*Chic.*), **25,** 49.

Namba, T. and Grob, D. (1971). Myasthenia gravis and hyperthyroidism occurring in two sisters. *Neurology* (*Minneap.*), **21,** 377.

Namba, T., Sato, T. and Grob, D. (1967). Myasthenia gravis. Serum globulin bound *in vivo* to skeletal muscle striations. *Arch. Neurol.* (*Chic.*), **17,** 637.

Oosterhuis, H. J. G. H. (1964). Studies in myasthenia gravis. I. A clinical study of 180 patients. *J. neurol. Sci.* (*Amst.*), **1,** 512.

Oosterhuis, H. J. G. H., Geld, H. Van Der and Feltkamp, T. E. W. (1967). Studies in myasthenia gravis. II. The relation of some clinical and immunological data. *J. neurol. Sci.*, **4,** 417.

Osserman, K. E. and Kaplan, L. I. (1953). Studies in myasthenia gravis. Use of edrophonium chloride (Tensilon) in differentiating myasthenic from cholinergic weakness. *Arch. Neurol. Psychiat.* (*Chic.*), **70,** 385.

Osserman, K. E. and Silver, S. (1961). The differential diagnosis of myopathy as seen in hyperthyroidism and myasthenia gravis. In "Advances in Thyroid Research". Edited by R. Pitt-Rivers, p. 100. Pergamon Press, Oxford.

Osserman, K. E., Tsairis, P. and Weiner, L. B. (1967). Myasthenia gravis and thyroid disease : clinical and immunologic correlation. *J. Mt. Sinai Hosp., N.Y.*, **34,** 469.

Pennington, G. W. and Wilson, A. (1961). Incidence of myasthenia gravis in the Merseyside conurbation. In "Myasthenia Gravis: the Second International Symposium Proceedings". Edited by H. R. Viets, p. 337. Thomas, Springfield, Illinois.

Ramsay, I. D. (1964). The Muscle Lesion in Thyrotoxicosis. M.D. Thesis. University of Edinburgh.

Ramsay, I. D. (1966). Muscle dysfunction in hyperthyroidism. *Lancet*, *ii*, 931.

Ramsay, I. D. (1967). Unpublished.

Ramsay, I. (1968). Thyrotoxic muscle disease. *Postgrad. med. J.*, **44,** 385.

Rapela, C. E. (1944). "Relacion de la Glandula Suprarenal Con el Timo." Edited by "El Atenco". Buenos Aires.

Reaves, L. E. (1965). Altered immunologic mechanisms in diseases of unknown cause: Report of myasthenia gravis, pernicious anaemia and myxedema occurring in the same patient. *Geriatrics*, **20,** 707.

Rennie, G. E. (1908). Exophthalmic goitre combined with myasthenia gravis. *Rev. Neurol. Psychiat.*, **6,** 229.

Ringertz, N. (1951). Pathology of the thymus and other organs in myasthenia gravis. *Acta path. microbiol. scand.*, **29,** 9.

Roitt, I. M. and Doniach, D. (1960). Thyroid auto-immunity. *Brit. med. Bull.*, **16,** 152.

Rowland, L. P., Aranow, H. Jr. and Hoefer, P. F. A. (1961). Current concepts of the pathogenesis of myasthenia gravis. *Internat. J. Neurol.*, **2,** 207.

Rowland, L. P., Aranow, H. Jr. and Hoefer, P. F. A. (1966). Endocrine aspects of myasthenia gravis. In "Progressive Muskeldystrophie, Myotonie, Myasthenie". Edited by E. Kuhn, p. 416. Springer-Verlag, Berlin.

Rowland, L. P., Hoefer, P. F. A. and Aranow, H. Jr. (1960). Myasthenic syndromes. *Res. Publ. Ass. nerv. ment. Dis.*, **28,** 548.

Russell, D. S. (1953). Histological changes in the striped muscles in myasthenia gravis. *J. Path. Bact.*, **65,** 279.

Sahay, B. M., Blendis, L. M. and Greene, R. (1965). Relation between myasthenia gravis and thyroid disease. *Brit. med. J.*, *i*, 762.

Sanderson, K. V. and Adey, W. R. (1952). Electromyographic and endocrine studies in chronic thyrotoxic myopathy. *J. Neurol. Neurosurg. Psychiat.*, **15,** 200.

Schimrick, K. (1966). Myasthenia gravis und Schilddrüse. In "Progressive Muskeldystrophie, Myotonie, Myasthenie". Vol. I. Edited by E. Kuhn, p. 426. Springer-Verlag, Berlin.

Schlezinger, N. S. and Corin, M. S. (1968). Myasthenia gravis associated with hyperthyroidism in childhood. *Neurology* (*Minneap.*), **18,** 1217.

Simpson, J. A. (1958). An evaluation of thymectomy in myasthenia gravis. *Brain*, **81,** 112.

Simpson, J. A. (1960). Myasthenia gravis: a new hypothesis. *Scot. med. J.*, **5,** 419.

Simpson, J. A. (1964). Immunological disturbances in myasthenia gravis with a report of Hashimoto's disease developing after thymectomy. *J. Neurol. Neurosurg. Psychiat.*, **27,** 485.

Simpson, J. A. (1966). Myasthenia gravis as an autoimmune disease: clinical aspects. *Ann. N.Y. Acad. Sci.*, **135,** 506.

Simpson, J. A. (1968). The correlations between myasthenia gravis and disorders of the thyroid gland. In "Research in Muscular Dystrophy". Proceedings IVth Symposium. Edited by members of the Research Committee of the Muscular Dystrophy Group, p. 31. Pitman Medical, London.

Simpson, J. A. (1969). In "Disorders of Voluntary Muscle". Edited by J. N. Walton, p. 555. Churchill, London.

Simpson, J. F., Westerberg, M. R. and Magee, K. R. (1966). Myasthenia gravis. An analysis of 295 cases. *Acta neurol. scand.*, **42,** Supp. 23.

Singer, W. and Sahay, B. M. (1966). Myasthenia gravis, Hashimoto's thyroiditis and pernicious anaemia. *Brit. med. J.*, *i*, 904.

Slomić, A., Rosenfalck, A. and Buchthal, F. (1968). Electrical and mechanical responses of normal and myasthenic muscle. *Brain Res.*, **10,** 1.

Storm-Mathisen, A. (1961). "Myasthenia Gravis." Aschehoug, Oslo, Almquist and Wiksell, Stockholm.

Sturgill, B. C., Carpenter, R. R., Strauss, A. J. L. and Goodman, H. C. (1964). Antibodies in systemic lupus erythematosus and myasthenia gravis which react with thermally denatured DNA-coated bentonite. *Proc. Soc. exp. Biol.*, **115,** 246.

Tabachnick, I. I. A., Thorstad, J. A., Wagner, J. and Parker, R. F. (1958). A partial pharmacologic profile of the response to neuromuscular blocking agents as modified by sodium L-thyroxine. *Arch. int. Pharmacodyn*, **114,** 210.

Thorn, G. W. and Eder, H. H. (1946). Studies on chronic thyrotoxic myopathy. *Amer. J. Med.*, **1,** 583.

Thorn, G. W. and Tierney, N. A. (1941). Myasthenia gravis complicated by thyrotoxicosis; creatine studies; case report. *Bull. Johns Hopk. Hosp.*, **69,** 469.

Thorner, M. W. (1939). Relation of myasthenia gravis to hyperthyroidism. *Arch. intern. Med.*, **64,** 330.

Van Der Geld, H., Feltkamp, T. E. W., Van Loghem, J. J., Oosterhuis, H. J. G. H. and Biemond, A. (1963). Multiple antibody production in myasthenia gravis. *Lancet*, *ii*, 373.

Van Der Geld, H., Feltkamp, T. E. W. and Oosterhuis, H. J. G. H. (1964). Reactivity of myasthenia gravis serum gamma globulin with skeletal muscle and thymus demonstrated by immunofluorescence. *Proc. Soc. Exp. Biol. Med.*, **115,** 782.

Van De Velde, R. *et al.* (1966). Quoted by Van Der Geld, H. W. R. and Strauss, A. J. L. (1966). "Myasthenia gravis: immunological relationship between striated muscle and thymus." *Lancet*, *i*, 57.

Verschuer, O. V. (1959). Die Zwillingsforschung im Dienste der inneren Medizin. *Verh. dtsh. Ges. inn. Med.*, **64,** 262.

Vetters, J. M. (1967). Muscle antibodies in myasthenia gravis. *Immunology*, **13,** 275.

Viets, H. R. and Schwab, R. S. (1935). Prostigmin in the diagnosis of myasthenia gravis. *New Engl. J. Med.*, **213,** 1280.

Warner, N. L. (1964). The immunological role of different lymphoid organs in the chicken. II. The immunological competence of thymic cell suspensions. *Aust. J. exp. Biol. med. Sci.*, **42,** 401.

Weigert, C. (1901). Pathologisch-anatomischer Beitrag zur Erbschen Krankheit (Myasthenia Gravis). *Neurol. Zbl.*, **20,** 597.

Werner, S. C. (1955). Euthyroid patients with early eye signs of Graves' disease; their responses to L-triiodothyronine and thyrotropin. *Amer. J. Med.*, **18,** 608.

White, R. G. and Marshall, A. H. E. (1962). The autoimmune response in myasthenia gravis. *Lancet*, *ii*, 120.

Whitfield, A. G. W. and Hudson, W. A. (1961). Chronic thyrotoxic myopathy. *Quart. J. Med.*, **30,** 257.

Wolf, S. M., Rowland, L. P., Schotland, D. L., McKinney, A. S., Hoefer, P. F. A. and Aranow, H. Jr., (1966). Myasthenia as an autoimmune disease: clinical aspects. *Ann. N.Y. Acad. Sci.*, **135,** 517.

Woolf, A. L. (1969). In "Disorders of Voluntary Muscle". Edited by J. N. Walton, pp. 221–228. Churchill, London.

Wright, R. and Kerr, J. H. (1967). Autoimmunity in myasthenia gravis: a family study. *Clin. exp. Immunol.*, **2,** 93.

Zaimis, E., Metaxas, N., Havard, C. W. H. and Campbell, E. D. R. (1965). Cardiovascular and skeletal muscle changes in cats treated with thyroxine. In "Researches in Muscular Dystrophy". Edited by Members of the Research Committee of the Muscular Dystrophy Group. Pitman Medical, London.

CHAPTER 3

THYROTOXIC PERIODIC PARALYSIS

Hypokalalaemic periodic paralysis is a rare syndrome which may occur either in the familial form, with autosomal dominant inheritance, or sporadically. Both forms of the disease are similar clinically and usually consist of intermittent attacks of weakness or actual muscle paralysis, associated in most instances with low serum potassium levels. As may be imagined, some of the sporadic cases have been associated with situations in which loss of potassium from the body occurs, such as primary aldosteronism, diuretic therapy, potassium-losing nephritis and renal tubular acidosis. However, a majority of the sporadic cases have occurred in patients with thyrotoxicosis.

Prevalence

Rosenfeld (1902) was the first to report the association of periodic paralysis with exophthalmic goitre. The first cases in the English literature were described by Dunlap and Kepler in 1931, but most subsequent reports came from Japan. By 1961, Engel noted that of 228 case reports of thyrotoxic periodic paralysis (T.P.P.) 90% were from Japan. In Japan thyrotoxicosis is frequently found among patients with periodic paralysis. In Itahara's (1961) series of 126 patients, 71 (56·3%) were found to have thyrotoxicosis. However, since then cases have been reported from Korea (Lee *et al.*, 1964; Kim and Cha, 1965), among both North and South Chinese living in Hong Kong (McFadzean and Yeung, 1967) and amongst the Japanese population of Hawaii (Okihiro and Beddow, 1965). A survey of the hospitals in Hawaii revealed that of 14 patients with sporadic periodic paralysis, 10 had thyrotoxicosis. Although only 29% of the population of Hawaii is Japanese, 9 out of the 10 patients were of that race, the tenth being an ethnic Hawaiian (Okihiro and Beddow, 1965). It therefore seems to be an undisputed fact that the disease is commonest among the Mongolian races of Japan and China.

Okinaka and his colleagues (1957) in Japan studied their 6333 thyrotoxic patients and found that 8·2% of the males and 0·4% of the females also had periodic paralysis. It might be argued that this prevalence* is falsely high since the only patients studied were ones admitted to hospital. Thus ambulatory patients who might have been less thyrotoxic were not included. Moreover, in 50% of cases the evidence for the presence of periodic paralysis depended entirely on the patient's history. However, another Japanese survey showed a similar overall prevalence of 8% amongst 432 thyrotoxic patients (Satoyoshi *et al.*, 1963a), while McFadzean and Yeung (1967) in Hong Kong discovered that of 1366 new thyrotoxic patients 13% of men and 0·17% of women gave a history of periodic paralysis. By comparison Hamfelt and Wetterberg (1964) found only one patient with periodic paralysis among 1202 thyrotoxic patients admitted to hospital in Sweden, although Linder (1955) somewhat surprisingly found 4 patients with periodic paralysis among 63 (6·3%) thyrotoxics treated at a New York hospital over a four-year period. The history seems to have been quite reliable in discovering the true prevalence of periodic paralysis in thyrotoxicosis, for of the 25 patients of McFadzean and Yeung (1967) who gave a positive history and were admitted to hospital, 8 developed spontaneous attacks while in hospital, 18 had attacks after induction with carbohydrate and insulin, and a further 5 after a similar induction, having been given 9α fluorohydrocortisone for three to five days beforehand.

The prevalence of periodic paralysis in thyrotoxic patients is far higher in men than women. Okinaka *et al.* (1957) found a male to female ratio of 20·5 to 1, compared with a ratio of 3 to 1 in patients with familial periodic paralysis. Engel (1961) in his review of 228 cases of thyrotoxic periodic paralysis calculated the male to female ratio as 6·6 to 1. In the survey of McFadzean and Yeung (1967) the ratio among Hong Kong Chinese was 11·5 to 1.

Unlike the uncomplicated form of periodic paralysis, a family history is not commonly obtained in the thyrotoxic patients. A positive family history was obtained in only 5 (2%) out of 228 cases (Engel, 1961). In 3 of the 5 patients, the affected relative also had thyrotoxicosis. Brown (1960) described the occurrence of periodic paralysis and thyrotoxicosis in three brothers.

In familial periodic paralysis (F.P.P.) more than 60% of the

* "Prevalence" is preferred to the frequently misused word "incidence", since in epidemiological terms the latter means the number of cases of a disease occurring per unit of population within a defined time interval (usually a year), whereas "prevalence" means the number of cases of a disease existing in a population at any given time.

patients have their first attack before the age of 16 (Talbott, 1941), whereas in only 8% of the thyrotoxics did the attacks begin before the age of 19, and in 84% the onset was between the ages of 20 and 39 (Engel, 1961). In both Okihiro and Beddow's (1965) Hawaiian and in McFadzean and Yeung's (1967) Chinese series the peak prevalence of thyrotoxic periodic paralysis was between the ages of 30 and 40. The age prevalence of thyrotoxic periodic paralysis in the Chinese patients coincided closely with that for uncomplicated hyperthyroidism (Fig. 3.1).

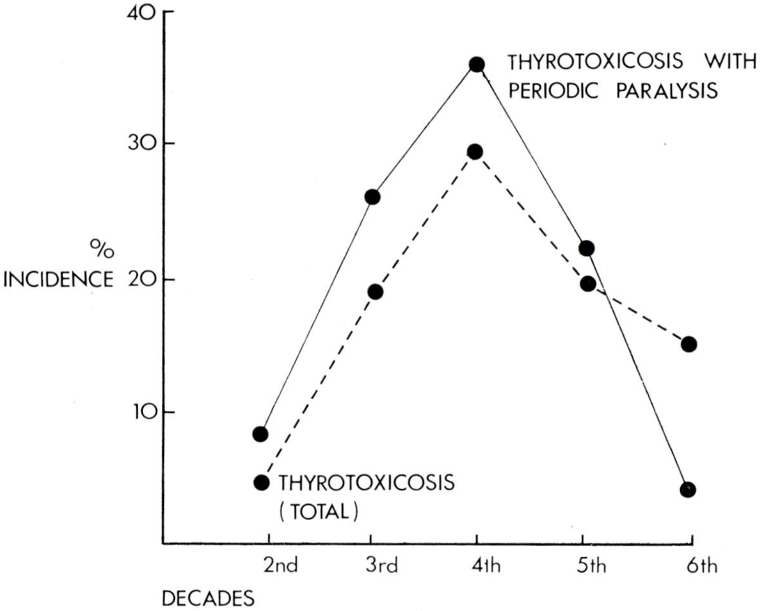

Figure 3.1. Age of onset, among Chinese males, of uncomplicated thyrotoxicosis (178 patients) compared with that of thyrotoxic periodic paralysis (23 patients). (From McFadzean and Yeung, 1967).

In a survey of the literature, Engel (1961) found that in 82% of cases the thyrotoxicosis preceded or appeared concurrently with the onset of attacks of periodic paralysis. In a prospective study carried out over a six-year period, McFadzean and Yeung (1967) concluded that the symptoms of thyrotoxicosis appeared from three months to nine years (mean 2·4 years) before the onset of periodic paralysis in 80% of their patients and that in the remaining 20% the onset of the two diseases was simultaneous.

Clinical features

Although the periodic paralysis is usually associated with Graves' disease, the hyperthyroidism may sometimes be due to an autonomous thyroid nodule (Norris, Clark and Biglieri, 1971).

In contrast to the commoner occurrence of attacks of familial periodic paralysis on wakening (McArdle, 1969), the attacks in thyrotoxic patients tend to come on in the evening or at night and rarely occur in the morning (Okinaka *et al.*, 1957; Satoyoshi *et al.*, 1963a; McFadzean and Yeung, 1967). The paralysis never occurs during exertion, but often happens while the patient is resting after exercise (Satoyshi *et al.*, 1963a; McFadzean and Yeung, 1967). McFadzean and Yeung found that some of their patients could "work off" an impending attack by starting to exercise once again.

Some patients noticed an aching or stiffness in the muscles affected before they became paretic (McFadzean and Yeung, 1967). The paralysis commonly affected proximal muscles of the legs first, then spread to arms and trunk, but spared extraocular muscles and muscles associated with breathing, talking and swallowing (Satoyoshi *et al.*, 1963a; McFadzean and Yeung, 1967). Usually patients with quite marked proximal muscle weakness were able to move their fingers and toes. Muscle involvement during an attack may vary from one simply of demonstrable clinical weakness to one of frank paralysis. McFadzean and Yeung (1967) found in induced attacks that during the early paretic stage the tendon jerks were enhanced and remained so well into the stage of complete paralysis, though later on both the tendon reflexes and the superficial reflexes were completely lost. At a stage of complete areflexic paralysis they noted the muscles were not flaccid, but were firm in consistence.

Some of McFadzean and Yeung's (1967) patients had asymmetrical paralysis and noticed that the muscles worst affected were those which had been used most during the previous bout of physical activity. When muscles of the pelvic girdle alone were affected, attacks tended to last for a few hours only, but if all muscles below the neck were involved, the attacks could go on for 48 hours. Satoyoshi *et al.* (1963a) observed one patient in whom the attacks lasted for as long as one week.

The frequency of attacks varies enormously. Satoyoshi *et al.* (1963a) found that the extremes were six attacks per week to two per year. Table 3.1 shows an analysis of the attack rates in 110 patients of Okinaka *et al.* (1957).

Other factors, apart from physical exertion, which have been

TABLE 3.1

Table showing the relative frequency of attacks of thyrotoxic periodic paralysis in a group of 110 Japanese patients (Okinaka et al., *1957)*

Frequency of attacks	No. of patients	%
> 1 every 2 weeks	43	39
1 every 1–2 months	21	19
1 every 6–12 months	46	42
Totals	110	100

noted to precipitate attacks of periodic paralysis are heavy carbohydrate meals and the ingestion of alcohol (Satoyoshi *et al.*, 1963a; McFadzean and Yeung, 1967). The Japanese and Chinese patients tended to have a high carbohydrate intake, particularly of rice, and this increased considerably following the onset of thyrotoxicosis, probably because of the greater appetite associated with that disease (McFadzean and Yeung, 1967). McFadzean and Yeung also remarked on the frequency of attacks among these patients during the summer months when the temperature in Hong Kong rises above 30°C, and there is high humidity and noted the rarity of attacks during the winter then the temperature falls to 20°C or below and there is less humidity. They pointed out that, during the summer, working people in Hong Kong slake their thirst with cold drinks, rich in sugar, a substance first noticed by Shinosaki (1926) to precipitate attacks. Satoyoshi and Kinoshita (1970) have noted that in recent years the incidence of thyrotoxic periodic paralysis has dropped in Japan. They attributed this to economic and nutritional improvements and to a consequent change in diet.

Muscular recovery from an attack of thyrotoxic periodic paralysis occurs in reverse order to the original sequence of spread and the time needed for full muscle strength to return is directly proportional to the severity and duration of the attack (McFadzean and Yeung, 1967).

Induction of attacks

McFadzean and Yeung (1967) were able to induce attacks of paralysis in 18 out of 23 patients with a history suggestive of the condition by giving 30 units of soluble insulin before a lunch containing 200 G of carbohydrate in the form of rice and a further 30 units of soluble insulin before an evening meal containing the same amount of carbohydrate. The patients were encouraged to take glucose drinks and to walk about during the afternoon and to retire to bed after the evening meal. The attacks of paralysis usually started three hours after the evening meal and reached their maximum after another two to four hours.

The 5 patients who did not have an attack while on this regime were all successfully induced by the same method after receiving 9α fluorohydrocortisone 0·6 mg/day for between three and five days. Conversely, 4 out of 8 patients who had been successfully induced initially did not have an attack of paralysis on the carbohydrate and insulin regime after being given 12 G of potassium chloride per day for five days before the attempt was made. In the 4 patients who did have an induced attack, despite being pre-treated with potassium chloride, spironolactone in a dosage of 200 mg per day for five days before a further attempt of precipitating paralysis, only prevented an attack in one patient, but studies of urinary potassium showed that spironolactone had not significantly reduced the excretion of this ion. In a further experiment, pre-treatment with potassium chloride as well as the spironolactone was unsuccessful in preventing induced paralysis.

Satoyoshi *et al.* (1963a) were able to bring on an attack of paralysis by giving acetazoleamide (Diamox) in a dosage of 200 mg per day for two days. This diuretic causes the loss of a significant amount of potassium in the urine. This is difficult to reconcile with the claim of Griggs, Engel and Resnick (1970) that acetazoleamide dramatically abolished attacks and improved inter-attack weakness in 10 out of 12 patients with familial periodic paralysis. In a patient with thyrotoxic periodic paralysis Norris, Clark and Biglieri (1971) believed that 600 mg of acetazoleamide per day prevented attacks over a 17-day period. In the study of Griggs, Engel and Resnick (1970) the acetazoleamide produced a mild metabolic acidosis but had no demonstrable effect on total body sodium or potassium.

The effect of thyroid hormone

Thyroid hormone appears to have different effects on the thyrotoxic and familial forms of periodic paralysis. Wolf (1943) found that in 7 patients with the familial form, the attacks could be prevented by the prior administration of thyroid extract. It is difficult to understand the mechanism since he used 3 grains of dried thyroid, which is the equivalent of 0·3 mg of L-thyroxine and represents a physiological dosage. Its only effect in the euthyroid subject should be to inhibit the secretion of thyroid stimulating hormone. One of Wolf's (1943) patients developed factitious thyrotoxicosis because of over-enthusiastic self-medication, but paralysis only returned when the thyroid was stopped.

Engel (1961) found that hypermetabolism induced in a patient with familial periodic paralysis by means of L-triiodothyronine or by thyroid stimulating hormone did not worsen the disease. However, exacerbations followed the withdrawal of both agents and were controlled by the readministration of thyroid stimulating hormone.

So far as the thyrotoxic form of periodic paralysis is concerned, alleviation of the hyperthyroidism nearly always gets rid of further attacks of paralysis. In a review of 159 cases in the literature, many of them followed up by a postal survey (Okinaka *et al.*, 1957), Engel (1961) found that the thyrotoxicosis was stated to be cured in 152 patients and ameliorated in a further 7; the periodic paralysis had been completely abolished in 141 patients and improved in 10 others.

In a more recent prospective study of 25 patients McFadzean and Yeung (1967) found no spontaneous attacks of paralysis occurring in the patients once they had been rendered euthyroid by whatever means. In 9 patients who had had frequent and severe attacks while thyrotoxic the authors were unable to induce attacks with a high carbohydrate intake and insulin as described previously. Four patients were given 9α fluorohydrocortisone 0·6 mg per day for five days before induction, but in each case it failed. The addition of physiological doses of triiodothyronine to the 9α fluorohydrocortisone made no difference. No patient developed paralysis. This inability to provoke attacks of paralysis in patients rendered euthyroid has also been noted by others (Linder, 1955; Overholt, Smith and White, 1957). Six patients who relapsed following withdrawal of their carbimazole therapy developed spontaneous attacks of paralysis early on, at a time when their symptoms of thyrotoxicosis were judged to be quite mild. This probably explains why some patients have been described (Satoyoshi *et al.*, 1963a) who appeared to have developed periodic paralysis before the onset of clinical thyrotoxicosis. The relationship between relapse of the thyrotoxicosis and the recurrence of attacks of paralysis has also been remarked upon by Dunlap and Kepler (1931), Seed (1947) and Okihiro and Beddow (1965).

A few cases of periodic paralysis have persisted despite seemingly

TABLE 3.2

*Motor unit analysis in thyrotoxic periodic paralysis (from Norris, 1966)**

	Pre-paralytic		Paralytic		Euthyroid, one year after radioactive iodine treatment
Deltoid muscle					
Mean action potential duration ± SE (msec.)	5·6 ± 0·9		5·3 ± 1·3	†	9·4 ± 0·9
Polyphasic potentials (%)	50		56		22
Mean action potential amplitude ± SE (mV)	1·13 ± 0·20	†	0·52 ± 0·25	†	1·22 ± 0·41
Dorsal interosseous muscle					
Mean action potential duration ± SE (msec.)	5·5 ± 1·1		5·2 ± 1·0	†	8·4 ± 1·5
Polyplasic potentials (%)	40		40		6
Mean action potential amplitude ± SE (mV)	0·61 ± 0·24		0·57 ± 0·21	†	1·32 ± 0·23

* 20–30 different motor unit action potentials measured in each case.
† Difference significant ($p < 0{\cdot}01$).

adequate control of the thyrotoxicosis (Dunlap and Kepler, 1931), but these exceptions are rare.

ELECTROMYOGRAPHY

Norris (1966), in a careful study of a thyrotoxic patient both between and during attacks of induced periodic paralysis, found no evidence of abnormalities in motor neurone excitability, peripheral nerve function or neuromuscular transmission. However, direct electrical stimulation of the quadriceps muscle produced normally strong contractions before and after an induced attack of paralysis, but not during an attack, when a 40–50% reduction in the amplitude of the evoked potentials took place. Table 3.2 shows the results of electromyography. There was evidence of a myopathy in the studies carried out on the deltoid and dorsal interosseous muscles both before and during an induced attack of paralysis, in that the mean action potential duration was reduced and the percentage of polyphasic potentials increased compared with the recordings taken a year later when the patient was euthyroid and attack-free. There were no significant differences in these parameters in the recordings taken before and during a paralytic attack. These E.M.G. findings are in keeping with those of thyrotoxicosis generally (Ramsay, 1965) and need not necessarily have anything to do with periodic paralysis. However, there was a significant reduction in mean action potential amplitude in the deltoid during an attack compared with previously, and this must be attributable to the paralysis.

Norris and his colleagues (1971) have recently performed electromyography on another patient with thyrotoxic periodic paralysis. There was no abnormal spontaneous activity except during the induction of hypoglycaemia. Once again there were decreases of the evoked action potential amplitudes in the vastus medialis and gastrocnemus. Rather unexpectedly there was an increase in the action potential amplitudes found in vastus medialis on minimal effort. Norris, Clark and Biglieri (1971) thought that this might indicate that the smaller motor units are more affected in thyrotoxic periodic paralysis, but this is difficult to reconcile with Norris' (1966) earlier findings. Brody and Dudley (1969) were unable to find any E.M.G. abnormalities in a patient studied between attacks.

ELECTROCARDIOGRAPHIC CHANGES

E.C.G. changes during both spontaneous and induced attacks have been studied by McFadzean and Yeung (1967). They invariably found patterns characteristic of hypokalaemia, even in patients who had attacks when the serum potassium level was within normal limits. Atrial and ventricular ectopic beats occurred frequently. Atrial fibrillation and paroxysmal supraventricular tachycardia were noted on one occasion each, but like the ectopic beats could be reversed by giving potassium intravenously. Prolongation of the P–R interval occurred in 27% of the attacks and 3 patients developed reversible right bundle-branch block. McFadzean and Yeung (1967) recommended that the induction of paralysis should only be carried out with the patient connected to a cardiac monitor and that intravenous potassium should be readily available.

BIOCHEMISTRY

Potassium and sodium

The most consistent change found in thyrotoxic periodic paralysis, as in the familial form, is a fall in the level of serum potassium. During maximal paralysis Satoyoshi *et al.* (1963a) found in 6 patients a reduction in serum potassium to a mean level of 2·77 m Eq/l. However, as the work of McFadzean and Yeung (1967) has shown, serum potassium levels, although falling during an attack, may remain within normal physiological levels. Figure 3.2 shows that the level was reduced to below the normal range in eight out of 13 spontaneous attacks, in 10 out of 18 carbohydrate and insulin-induced attacks, and in four out of five attacks induced after pre-treatment with 9α fluorohydrocortisone. In the patients given either spironolactone alone or spironolactone and potassium chloride together before induction, the serum potassium levels remained within normal limits. It was noted, though, that the paralysis was more severe and extensive among those with the lowest potassium levels. In a recent study of one patient Norris, Clark and Biglieri (1971) found a poor correlation between the fall in serum potassium and the degree of paralysis. Moreover, the clinical attack cleared without the serum potassium level rising.

Serum electrolytes in between attacks have been found to be normal, with the exception of sodium which was slightly lower than in controls (Satoyoshi *et al.*, 1963a). On days when paralysis occurred there was a reduction in the excretion of water, sodium and potassium in the urine, but no excessive loss of potassium occurred in between attacks (McFadzean and Yeung, 1967). Aldosterone can probably be ruled out as an aetiological agent in the induction of paralysis since the urinary excretion of the hormone was normal and there was no upset in sodium balance (Norris, Panner and Stormont, 1968;

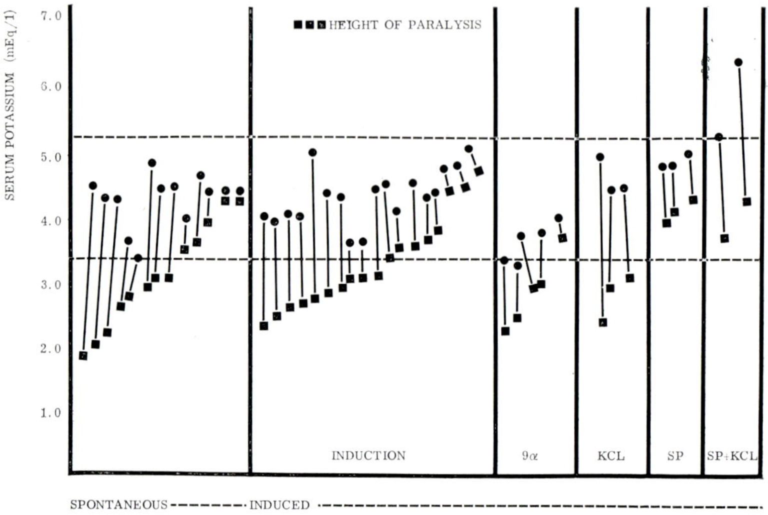

Figure 3.2. Changes in serum potassium concentration during spontaneous and induced attacks of thyrotoxic periodic paralysis. The normal range lies between the horizontal lines. Induction = induction with insulin and carbohydrate. 9α = induction after treatment with 9α fluorohydrocortisone. KCL = successful induction despite the prior administration of potassium chloride. Sp = successful induction despite the prior administration of spironolactone. Sp + KCL = successful induction despite the prior administration of both potassium chloride and spironolactone. (From McFadzean and Yeung, 1967).

Norris, Clark and Biglieri, 1971), though Shizume and his colleagues (1966b) did find an increase in exchangeable sodium in T.P.P.

Satoyoshi and his colleagues (1963a) measured serial electrolytes, haematocrit, haemoglobin, serum proteins and serum water in 4 patients before and during an induced attack of thyrotoxic periodic paralysis. The results were similar in the 4 patients and Fig. 3.3 illustrates the course of events in one of them. It can be seen that the basic initial change was an increase in serum water with a consequent dilution of the other constituents. As the paralysis started and progressed a reverse process took place with resulting haemoconcentration.

Shizume *et al.* (1966a) did a comparative study on patients with familial periodic paralysis and on patients with thyrotoxic periodic paralysis. They found a constant positive arteriovenous difference

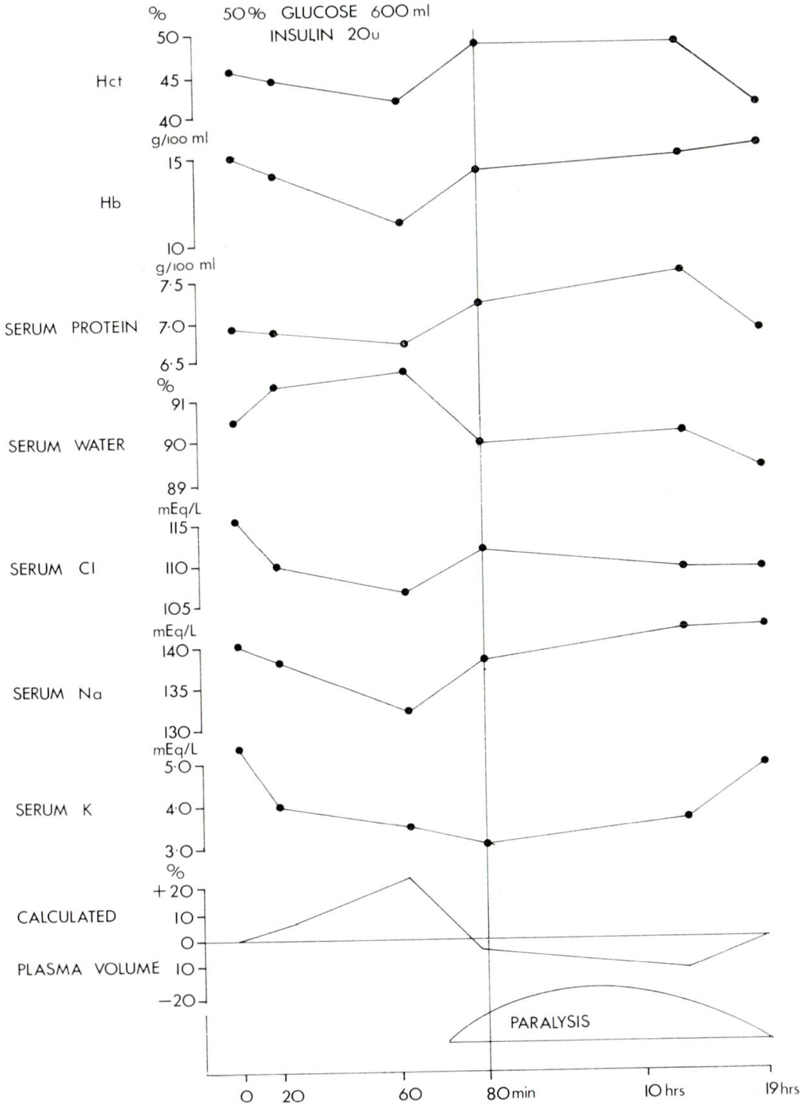

Figure 3.3. Alterations in blood and serum constituents during an attack of periodic paralysis induced in a thyrotoxic patient by the administration of glucose and insulin. (From Satoyoshi *et al.*, 1963a.)

for potassium in the leg during paralysis in both groups of patients. Total body potassium measured during attack-free intervals was lower than normal in the thyrotoxics. When the total body potassium was related to lean body mass it was found to be reduced, compared to controls, but not significantly so (Shizume *et al.*, 1966b). There was no statistical difference between the total exchangeable potassium/kg lean body mass in patients with thyrotoxic periodic paralysis and in uncomplicated hyperthyroidism (Shizume *et al.*, 1966b). Perhaps if the number of patients with thyrotoxic periodic paralysis had been greater the figures for K^e/kg lean body mass might have become significant statistically.

In the patients with idiopathic familial paralysis there was a very definite reduction in total exchangeable potassium whether it was related to body weight or lean body mass (Shizume *et al.*, 1966b). Exchangeable sodium was normal in this group of patients but significantly increased in the patients with thyrotoxic periodic paralysis. The authors postulated that the most likely mechanism for the production of both types of hypokalaemic periodic paralysis was some transient alteration of cell membrane permeability to potassium and/or sodium. Green and Matty (1962) have already shown that increased permeability of membranes to water can be induced by excess thyroid hormone.

Shizume and his co-workers (Shishiba *et al.*, 1966) followed up these total exchangeable potassium studies with muscle biopsies. They found that the potassium content of muscle and the intracellular concentrations of potassium were moderately reduced in patients with familial periodic paralysis compared with normals. The intracellular potassium content in thyrotoxic patients without paralysis was normal, as has been found by Staffurth and Thompson (1965), though total body exchangeable potassium studies did suggest that there was a general depletion in body potassium.

However, Shizume and his colleagues (Shishiba *et al.*, 1966) found that the ratio of intracellular to extracellular potassium concentration before the induction of paralysis was significantly higher in patients with T.P.P. than in patients with thyrotoxicosis alone. When attacks of paralysis were induced in T.P.P. there was a reduction in extracellular potassium concentration, more marked in those with the most severe paralysis, but little change in the intracellular concentration. Despite this, there was a very good correlation between the increase in the intracellular to extracellular potassium ratio and the severity of the paralysis.

Satoyoshi *et al.* (1963a) were able to obtain muscle biopsies in

6 thyrotoxic patients between attacks and in 4 patients during an attack. The intracellular and extracellular water of muscle was within the normal range in between attacks of paralysis and did not change significantly during an attack, though Norris, Clark and Biglieri (1971) noted a small but significant increase in muscle water content during induced paralysis. Between attacks intracellular potassium content expressed per 100 G of solid tissue was normal; during attacks the values fell but not significantly (Satoyoshi *et al.*, 1963a). On the other hand the potassium concentration expressed per litre of intracellular water did fall to a statistically significantly low level during an attack of paralysis. The intracellar sodium levels were double the normal values and fell to normal during an attack. Shy *et al.* (1961) were unable, in patients with familial periodic paralysis, to demonstrate abnormal muscle levels of sodium and potassium during an attack.

Magnesium and calcium

Recently Ishigami and his colleagues (1971) have studied magnesium levels in periodic paralysis. They found a constant fall in serum potassium and a rise in magnesium during an attack. The more marked were the changes, the more severe the paralysis. In patients with thyrotoxic periodic paralysis treatment of the hyperthyroidism prevented induced attacks of paralysis and during the attempt the changes in serum potassium and magnesium were minimal. The significance of this finding is as yet unknown, but it should be remembered that magnesium competes with calcium for receptor sites in muscle which are important in the acetylcholine-induced initiation of muscle contraction (Del Castillo and Katz, 1954a, b).

Engel and Lambert (1969) have recently studied the effect of adding calcium to muscle fibres obtained by biopsy from patients with familial hypokalaemic periodic paralysis during an attack. Calcium delivered directly to the myofilament space was found to activate the contractile mechanism of electrically inexcitable muscle. They thought therefore, that the failure of excitation–contraction coupling in periodic paralysis must lie in the fibre membranes. Since the sarcoplasmic reticulum was dilated during the attack they postulated that the prime fault lay in the release of calcium rather than in its uptake. Brody and Dudley (1969) found that the uptake of calcium by a microsomal fraction of muscle from a patient with thyrotoxic periodic paralysis was normal.

MISCELLANEOUS BIOCHEMICAL CHANGES

(Satoyoshi et al., 1963a)

Muscle inorganic phosphorus, creatine phosphate and adenosine triphosphate (ATP) were found to be normal in between attacks of T.P.P. One patient, who also had a biopsy while he was paralysed, had normal levels of inorganic phosphorus, but creatine phosphate and ATP had fallen to half the non-paralytic values.

Serum levels of aldolose and lactic dehydrogenase were normal in between attacks of T.P.P. though that of creatine phosphokinase was elevated. During an attack, however, levels of all three enzymes increased abruptly. Intramuscular enzyme levels were measured in one patient and these showed a reduction of all three during an attack to about a half of the previous values.

Carbohydrate metabolism

Glucose intolerance has been found in 3 patients with thyrotoxic periodic paralysis (Norris, Panner and Stormont, 1968; Hofmann and Smith, 1970; Norris, Clark and Biglieri, 1971). It may be of no aetiological importance since many thyrotoxic patients show this change, though Norris (1962) found it in familial periodic paralysis also.

It has been suggested that in the familial type of periodic paralysis there may be a block at the hexose phosphate stage of carbohydrate metabolism, alteration of pyruvate and lactate exchange and deficiency of co-carboxylase (McArdle, 1956; Shy *et al.*, 1961; Satoyoshi, Suzuki and Abe, 1963b). However, Engel and his associates (1967) were unable to find any abnormality in the synthesis of glycogen and could demonstrate no accumulation of intermediate products of glycolysis in muscle taken from a patient during an attack. This is in keeping with the finding by Norris, Clark and Biglieri (1971) of similar quantities of glycogen in the muscle fibres of their thyrotoxic patient both before and during attacks of paralysis.

MEMBRANE POTENTIALS

Shy and his colleagues (1961) found a normal resting potential of the muscle fibres *in vivo* during an attack of periodic paralysis of the familial type. However, the fibre was unable to conduct a propagated potential when stimulated. Hofmann and Smith (1970) have recently studied a Japanese-Hawaiian patient with thyrotoxic periodic paralysis and two others with familial periodic paralysis. Muscle biopsies were obtained from the intercostal muscles and compared *in vitro* with controls. All the specimens from the patients were significantly depolarized compared to controls and thus appeared abnormally sensitive to isolation. Further depolarization took place in the patients' fibres under the influence of insulin when the concentration of potassium in the bathing medium was normal, but strongly repolarized when the potassium was reduced to zero. Normal fibres in a potassium free medium were depolarized by insulin.

Removal of 90% of the sodium from the bathing fluid restored the resting mean potential of the diseased fibres to normal, but excitability was not restored. Increasing the concentration of calcium four-fold in the bathing medium partly restored the resting mean potential in both the thyrotoxic and the familial form of the paralysis: Procaine, an agent which "stabilizes" membranes by reducing the permeability to sodium (Shanes, 1958), partly restored both the resting mean potentials and the ability of the fibres to contract. Hofmann and Smith (1970) found increased amounts of sodium and decreased potassium in the fibres of both types of paralysis. They felt it unlikely that potassium movement was of any great importance in the induction of attacks of paralysis, but that abnormal sodium permeability of the fibre membrane might be. Norris and his colleagues (1971) have commented that the choice of intercostal muscle, rarely involved in paralysis, must lead one to reserve judgement on the significance of Hofmann and Smith's (1970) results.

MUSCLE PATHOLOGY

Light microscopy

Muscle biopsies taken from patients with thyrotoxicosis in between attacks of periodic paralysis have either been normal or have shown very minor degenerative changes (Satoyoshi *et al.*, 1963a; Jackman and Jones, 1964; Engel, 1966b; Norris, Panner and Stormont, 1968; Norris, Clark and Biglieri, 1971). Biopsies taken during an induced attack have occasionally shown no abnormality (Robertson, 1954; Engel, 1966b), but more usually have shown distinct alterations in structure. The most frequent finding is one of central and subsarcolemmal vacuoles, between 1 and 15 μ in diameter, some extending over several sarcomeres (Norris, Panner and Stormont, 1968; Brody and Dudley, 1969; Bergman *et al.*, 1970a; Norris, Clark and Biglieri, 1971). These vacuoles are indistinguishable from those seen in familial paralysis (Shy *et al.*, 1961). Brody and Dudley (1969) found that many fibres contained subsarcolemmal accumulations of P.A.S.-

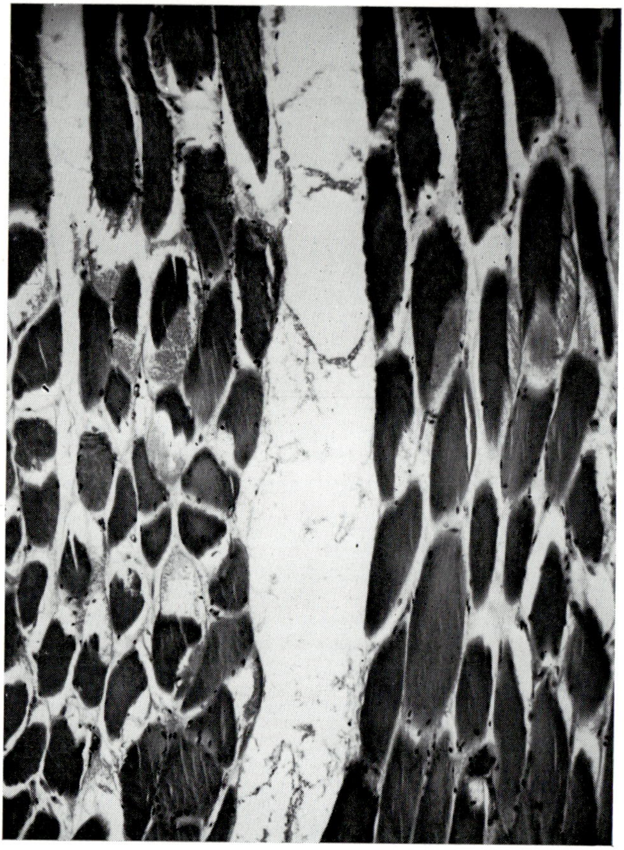

Figure 3.4. Transverse and tangential sections (×100) showing subsarcolemmal masses of P.A.S.-positive material in the shape of "half moons". (From Brody and Dudley, 1969.)

positive material which looked like half-moons on transverse section (Fig. 3.4) and were similar to those described in thyroid and pituitary disease by workers in Asböe-Hansen's laboratory (Asböe-Hansen, Iversen and Wichmann, 1952; Iversen, Asböe-Hansen and Carlsen, 1953; Kirchheiner, 1962). Similar accumulations have been found in 2 patients with thyrotoxic myopathy by Engel (1966a). The accumulations were susceptible to the actions of diastase and hyaluronidase and appeared to consist of glycogen (Brody and Dudley, 1969).

Bergman and his colleagues (1970a) pointed out that all these light microscopic data have been obtained by the study of 5 to 10 μ paraffin sections. This means that only major structural alterations will be seen. Electron microscopy on the other hand will cause

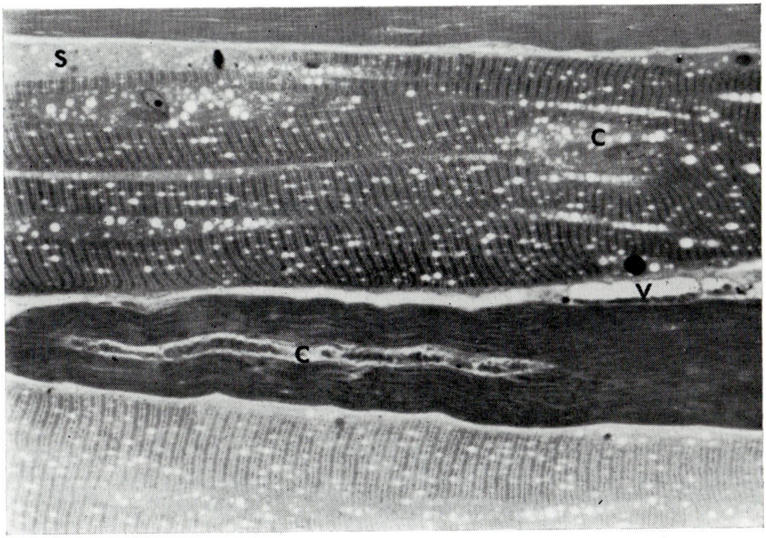

Figure 3.5. Quadriceps biopsy taken from a patient with thyrotoxic periodic paralysis in between attacks. Longitudinal section (×400; toluidine blue) showing amorphous subsarcolemmal lesions containing vacuoles (S). There are several central perinuclear lesions with myofibrillar breakdown and small vacuoles (c). The fibres contain numerous small vacuoles. V indicates a peripheral sarcolemmal blob. (From Bergman *et al.*, 1970a.)

pathological abnormalities to be missed because of the small area of tissue being examined. They thought that these difficulties could be overcome by the use of 1 μ sections of plastic embedded tissue. Using this method they described changes on light microscopy which had not been seen by other workers. In addition to the vacuolated areas already mentioned they found that many fibres contained hyalinized areas, sometimes vacuolated, which were mainly central in situation and which represented the breakdown of myofibrils (Fig. 3.5). Occasional central and subsarcolemmal accumulations of amorphous material were often found (Fig. 3.6). Occasional fibres were seen which had completely degenerated and were filled with vacuoles and lysosomes (Fig. 3.7). Some showed encroachment of the sarcolemma by amorphous material from other fibres (Fig. 3.7). Many fibres showed an increase in their intermyofibrillar spaces

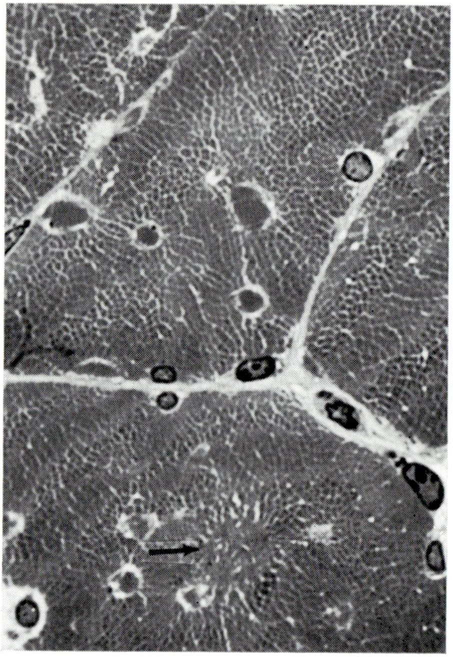

Figure 3.6. Same patient as in Fig. 3.5. Cross section at high magnification (×1000; toluidine blue) showing collections of amorphous material. The arrow indicates another type of lesion which probably signifies myofibrillar disarray. (From Bergman *et al.*, 1970a.)

which were filled with a P.A.S.-positive substance, probably glycogen (Fig. 3.8). In contrast, the control and subsarcolemmal vacuoles and the amorphous areas were not P.A.S.-positive. Nor were the myofibrils. Thus there did not seem to be any evidence of glycogen accumulation in the muscles of this patient with thyrotoxic periodic paralysis, though it should be noted that the biopsy was taken

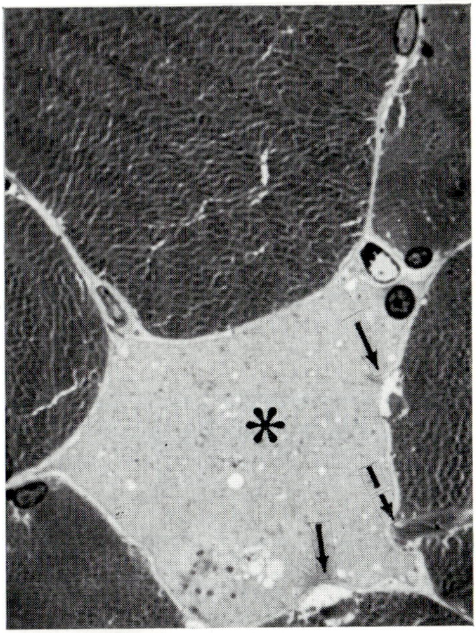

Figure 3.7(a). Same patient as in Fig. 3.5 (×1000; toluidine blue). The star indicates a degenerated fibre devoid of myofibrils but containing small vacuoles. Vacuolar lesions with amorphous material within them protrude from neighbouring fibres (arrows). (From Bergman *et al*., 1970a.)

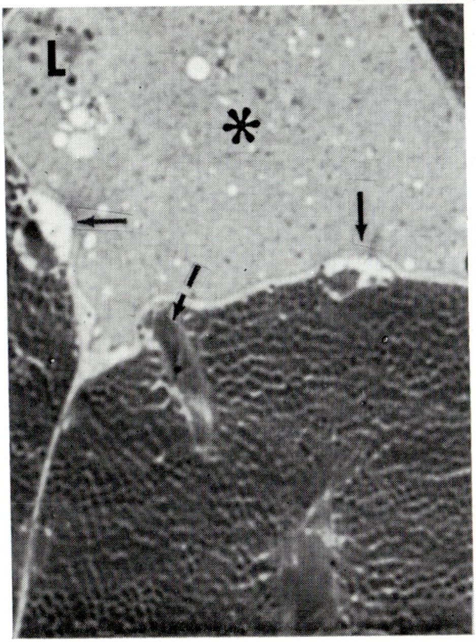

Figure 3.7(b). Higher magnification of Fig. 3.7(*a*). There is a collection of lysosomes (L) in a fibre devoid of myofibrils (star). The arrows indicate the same amorphous material as in Fig. 3.7(*a*). (From Bergman *et al*., 1970a.)

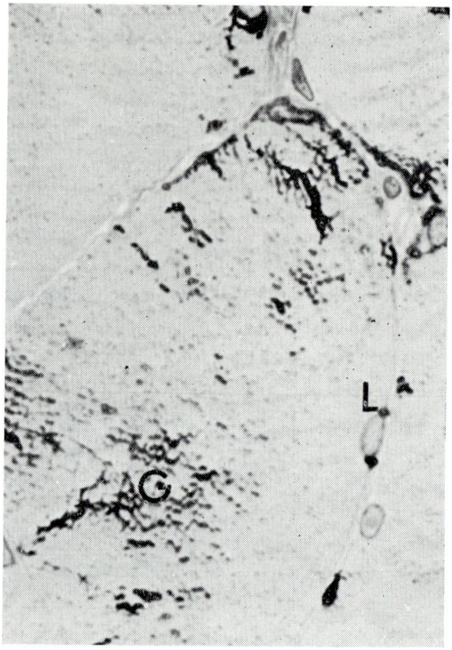

Figure 3.8. Same patient as in Fig. 3.5. There is PAS-positive material, probably glycogen (G), within an enlarged intermyofibrillar space. Two perinuclear lysosomes (L) are seen. (×1500; P.A.S.). (From Bergman *et al.*, 1970a)

during an attack-free interval. The muscle spindles seemed to be normal. The nuclei were variable in shape, some being oval and others round, but large nucleoli were usually present. Nuclear chains were only encountered once.

Electron microscopy

In recent years several electron microscopic studies have been carried out on the skeletal muscles of thyrotoxic patients both before and during induced attacks of paralysis (Engel, 1966b; Norris, Panner and Stormont, 1968; Brody and Dudley, 1969; Bergman *et al.*, 1970b; Cheah and Kan, 1971; Norris, Clark and Biglieri, 1971).

Some of the vacuoles, already noted on light microscopy, were found to extend over several sarcomeres (Fig. 3.9). At high magnification the larger vacuoles were not limited by any membrane other than those of the smaller vacuoles surrounding them (Fig. 3.9). Bergman and his colleagues (1970b) found the vacuoles in close association with myofibrils, lipid accumulations and tubular arrays, the latter often having dense membrane bound particles near them (Fig. 3.10).

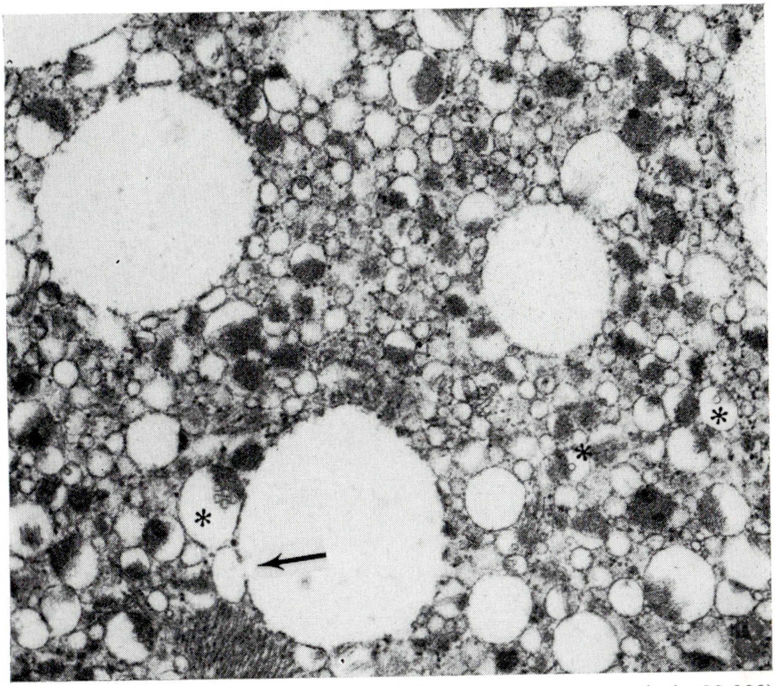

Figure 3.9. Same patient as in Fig. 3.5. Electron micrograph (×33,000) of a cross section showing how the accumulation of small vacuoles and membrane-bound particles and their subsequent fusion may lead to large vacuole formation (arrow). Within the membranous sacs (*) tubules 300A in diameter may be seen. (From Bergman *et al.*, 1970b.)

Brody and Dudley (1969) discovered that the subsarcolemmal "half-moons" seen on light microscopy were composed of dense aggregates of glycogen and mitochondria. These findings have recently been confirmed by Cheah and Kan (1971). Glycogen was also seen in the interfibrillar spaces (Cheah and Kan, 1971; Norris, Clark and Biglieri, 1971), but since Norris and his colleagues (1971)

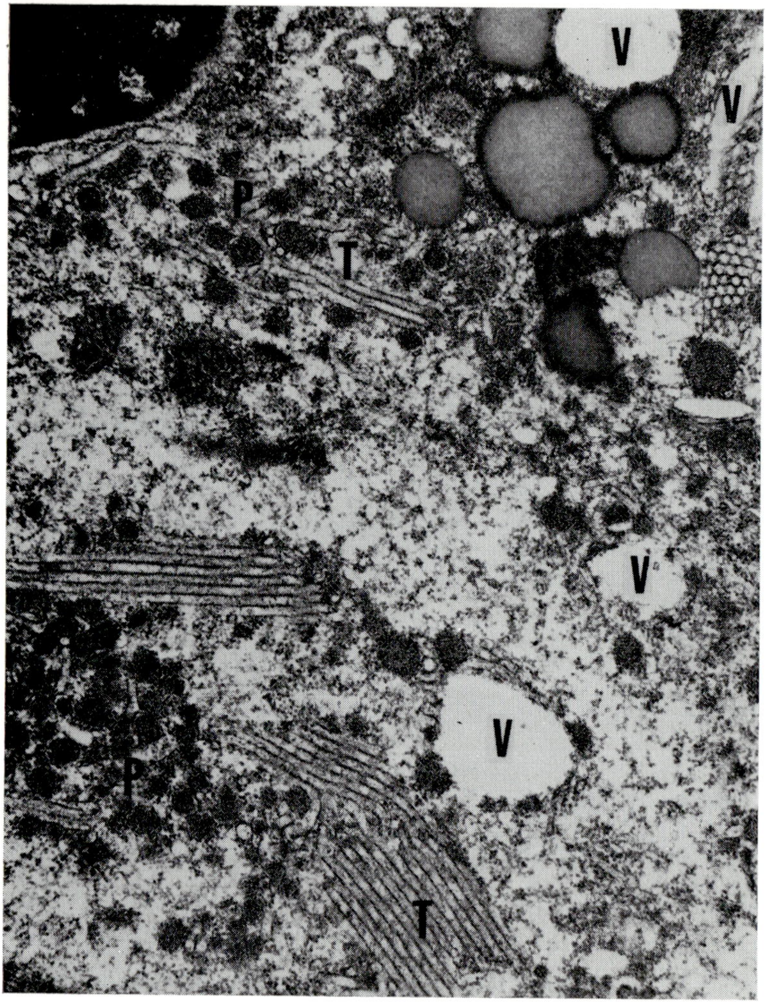

Figure 3.10. Same patient as in Fig. 3.5. Electron micrograph (×20,000) showing the relationship between tubular aggregates (T), membrane-bound particles (P) and vacuoles (V). (From Bergman *et al.*, 1970b.)

found the same amount of glycogen in the pre-paralytic and paralytic muscle specimens they concluded that it was possibly not important.

During an attack of paralysis the interfibrillar spaces became widened and fluid accumulated under the sarcolemma and elements of the sarcoplasmic reticulum became dilated (Norris, Clark and Biglieri, 1971).

The dilatations in the sarcotubular system noted by Engel (1966b) and by Norris, Panner and Stormont (1968) may have nothing to do with periodic paralysis since they were also found in thyrotoxic myopathy (Engel, 1966a). Similarly, the degenerative changes (Norris, Panner and Stormont, 1968; Schutta and Armitage, 1969b; Bergman *et al.*, 1970b) may be attributed to the general effects of thyrotoxicosis on muscle (Norris, Clark and Biglieri, 1971).

The most constant finding has been that of vacuolization which is present between attacks, but greatly increases during paralytic episodes. The degree of vacuolization does not seem to differ from that found in familial hypokalaemic periodic paralysis (Bergman *et al.*, 1970b).

Aetiology

In both the familial and the thyrotoxic forms of periodic paralysis the gross biochemical changes seem to be similar, namely a retention of sodium, water and potassium during an attack with a movement of potassium into muscle (Grob, Johns and Liljestrand, 1957; Shishiba *et al.*, 1966; Shizume *et al.*, 1966a, b). The attacks can also be precipitated in the same way by glucose and insulin. There, however, the similarity stops. Whereas in the case of familial periodic paralysis there is evidence of autosomal dominant inheritance (Sagild and Helweg-Larsen, 1955), it is exceptionally rare to find any family history among patients with the thyrotoxic form, apart from a few patients (Brown, 1960). Moreover, the age of onset is much later in the thyrotoxic patients and the age of onset was very close in McFadzean and Yeung's (1967) series to that of uncomplicated thyrotoxicosis. A further difference is in the response to thyroid medication. Whereas in thyrotoxic periodic paralysis it has an adverse effect (Shinosaki, 1926; Robertson, 1954), this does not seem to be true for the familial type and Wolf (1943) has even claimed that thyroid extract was beneficial in this condition. Indeed, Engel (1961) made one patient with familial period paralysis hypermetabolic with triiodothyronine and with thyroid stimulating hormone. On both occasions exacerbations of the disease took place only after cessation of the drug and while the basal metabolic rate was returning to normal.

Although attacks can usually be induced by glucose and insulin in the familial form, this is not possible once the thyrotoxic patient has been rendered euthyroid (McFadzean and Yeung, 1967). Thus, although Shinosaki's (1926) original suggestion that thyrotoxicosis unmasks a latent tendency to familial periodic paralysis is an attractive one, it does not seem to fit with the facts.

Satoyoshi and his colleagues (1963b) investigated carbohydrate metabolism in patients with the hypokalaemic form of periodic paralysis, including two patients with T.P.P. In the non-paralytic state they found elevated levels of lactate and pyruvate in the blood and lowered amounts of co-carboxylase (thiamine). Intensive thiamine treatment in these patients reduced the frequency and severity of spontaneous attacks and prevented the provocation of attacks by glucose and insulin. They thought that the disturbance in metabolism lay at the level of the oxidation of pyruvate to acetyl co-enzyme A. McFadzean and Yeung (1967) were, however, unable to show that the administration of thiamine to Hong Kong Chinese with thyrotoxic periodic paralysis had any effect.

A striking feature of thyrotoxic periodic paralysis is its predilection for men. Whereas uncomplicated thyrotoxicosis occurs four times as commonly in Japanese women as men, thyrotoxic periodic paralysis occurs five times as often in men as in women (Okinaka *et al.*, 1957). This suggests that the tendency for men to develop periodic paralysis is due either to an effect of testosterone or to a sex-linked gene. In support of the former is a report by Robertson (1954) of a doctor who took stilboestrol, in spite of the usual side effects, because it helped to prevent or ameliorate his attacks of paralysis.

The pathophysiological mechanism for the production of paralytic attacks remains unknown. Attacks are precipitated by physical exertion and by large carbohydrate meals (Satoyoshi *et al.*, 1963a, b; McFadzean and Yeung, 1967). Similarly they can be induced by the administration of glucose and insulin (McFadzean and Yeung, 1967). In both there is a fall in the serum potassium. During attacks of paralysis there is a reduction in the excretion of water, sodium and potassium in the urine (McFadzean and Yeung, 1967). Satoyoshi and his colleagues (1963a) showed that during an attack there was an increase in serum water with a consequent dilution of sodium and potassium. There is a conflict of evidence as to what happens to intracellular water during an attack of paralysis. Satoyoshi *et al.* (1963a) found no increase during attacks in 4 patients, but Norris and his colleagues (1971) showed small but significant increases in their study of one patient.

Although it is well known that the serum potassium falls during an attack, it is difficult to understand where the potassium goes, unless the apparent fall is produced by dilution. Satoyoshi *et al.* (1963a) even found that intracellular potassium levels fell during an attack. It seems likely therefore that changes in the movement of potassium ions are not the cause of the attacks of paralysis.

Much has been made of the presence of vacuoles in the paretic muscles. These have been interpreted as dilatations of the sarcoplasmic reticulum (Shy *et al.*, 1961; Engel, 1966b; Norris, Panner and Stormont, 1968). It is believed that the sarcoplasmic reticulum initiates myofibrillar contraction by releasing calcium ions (Winegrad, 1965) and relaxation by reaccumulating them (Weber, Herz and Reiss, 1963). Schutta and Armitage (1969b) thought that granular material which was distending the terminal sacs of the sarcoplasmic reticulum was calcium and that this might indicate a failure of calcium exchange between the sarcoplasmic reticulum and the myofibrils. Engel and Lambert (1969) showed that in F.P.P. calcium delivered directly to the myofilament space could initiate the contraction of electrically inexcitable muscle. They postulated that the primary fault lay in the release of calcium by the sarcoplasmic reticulum. Certainly Brody and Dudley's (1969) finding of a normal uptake of calcium by the sarcoplasmic reticulum in T.P.P. does not negate this hypothesis, and recent observations by Au and Yeung (1972) suggest that there is indeed an abnormality of the calcium pump in thyrotoxic periodic paralysis. They found that both the calcium pump adenosine triphosphatase activity and the total amount of calcium uptake by the sarcoplasmic reticulum showed a decrease during thyrotoxic periodic paralysis. Both these abnormalities reverted to normal after the attack. Au and Yeung (1972) thought that thyrotoxicosis might unmask latent periodic paralysis because it depletes ATP.

In addition to any changes in the sarcoplasmic reticulum, it seems likely that there is a disorder of muscle membrane excitability. Norris and his colleagues have shown a reduced amplitude of the evoked potential during attacks (Norris, 1966; Norris, Clark and Biglieri, 1971). Resting membrane potentials have been found to be normal in F.P.P., yet the fibre was unable to conduct a propagated action potential when stimulated (Shy *et al.*, 1961). Hofmann and Smith (1970) showed depolarization *in vitro* of muscle fibres from both F.P.P. and T.P.P. patients when exposed to insulin. They found that procaine, which stabilizes membranes by reducing sodium permeability (Shanes, 1958), partly restored resting membrane potentials and the contractility of the fibres to normal. This might suggest that an increase of membrane permeability to sodium is important in T.P.P. However, the exact abnormality of sarcolemmal function in T.P.P. remains as yet unknown.

Since the paralytic attacks come on quite rapidly it would seem that they are brought about by some metabolic change. Any neural effect seems to have been excluded (Norris, 1966; Norris, Clarke and Biglieri, 1971). The association of attacks with carbohydrate meals and exercise and the induction of attacks by glucose and insulin point to some abnormality of carbohydrate metabolism as being the initial trigger of the paralytic attacks in thyrotoxic patients. A profitable line of enquiry might be a comparative study of pancreatic insulin secretion and muscle glucose uptakes in thyrotoxic patients with and without periodic paralysis.

Treatment. Patients with thyrotoxic periodic paralysis should avoid a high carbohydrate intake and excessive exercise until they have been made euthyroid. There is evidence to suggest that large doses of potassium chloride (12 G per day in McFadzean and Yeung's series (1967)) may prevent attacks of paralysis. The aldosterone antagonist spironolactone was not found to be an effective prophylactic in the majority of patients (McFadzean and Yeung, 1967) and the usefulness of acetazolamide in a dosage of 600 mg per day (Norris, Clark and Biglieri, 1971) remains to be confirmed. Once an attack of paralysis has occurred the administration of potassium probably does nothing to shorten the length of the attack.

REFERENCES

Asböe-Hansen, G., Iversen, K. and Wichmann, R. (1952). Malignant exophthalmos: muscular changes and thyrotropin content in serum. *Acta endocr.*, **11,** 376.

Au, K.-S. and Yeung, R. T. T. (1972). Thyrotoxic periodic paralysis. Periodic variation in the muscle calcium pump activity. *Arch. Neurol.* (*Chic.*), **26,** 543.

Bergman, R. A., Afifi, A. K., Dunkle, L. M. and Johns, R. J. (1970a). Muscle pathology in hypokalaemic periodic paralysis with hyperthyroidism. I. High resolution light microscopic study of a case. *Johns Hopk. med. J.*, **126,** 88.

Bergman, R. A., Afifi, A. K., Dunkle, L. M. and Johns, R. J. (1970b). Muscle pathology in hypokalaemic paralysis with hyperthyroidism. II. A light and electron misroscopic study. *Johns Hopk. med. J.*, **126,** 100.

Brody, I. A. and Dudley, A. W. Jr. (1969). Thyrotoxic hypokalaemic periodic paralysis. Muscle morphology and functional assay of sarcoplasmic reticulum. *Arch. Neurol.* (*Chic.*), **21,** 1.

Brown, D. W. (1960). Periodic paralysis associated with hyperthyroidism in three brothers. *Hawaii med. J.*, **19,** 641.

Cheah, J. S. and Kan, S. P. (1971). Ultrastructure of the skeletal muscles in thyrotoxic periodic paralysis. *Aust. N. Z. J. Med.*, **3,** 250.

Del Castillo, J. and Katz, B. (1954a). The effect of magnesium on the activity of motor nerve endings. *J. Physiol.*, **124,** 553.

Del Castillo, J. and Katz, B. (1954b). Changes in end-plate activity produced by pre-synaptic polarization. *J. Physiol.*, **124,** 586.

Dunlap, H. F. and Kepler, E. J. (1931). Occurrence of periodic paralysis in course of exophthalmic goiter. *Proc. Mayo Clin.*, **6,** 272.

Engel, A. G. (1961). Thyroid function and periodic paralysis. *Amer. J. Med.*, **30,** 327.

Engel, A. G. (1966a). Electron microscopic observations in thyrotoxic and cortico-steroid induced myopathies. *Mayo Clin. Proc.*, **41,** 785.

Engel, A. G. (1966b). Electron microscopic observations in primary hypokalaemic and thyrotoxic periodic paralysis. *Mayo Clin. Proc.*, **41,** 797.

Engel, A. G. and Lambert, E. H. (1969). Calcium activation of electrically inexcitable muscle fibers in primary hypokalaemic periodic paralysis. *Neurology* (*Minneap.*), **19,** 851.

Engel, A. G., Potter, C. S. and Rosevear, J. W. (1967). Studies on carbohydrate metabolism and mitochondrial respiratory activities in primary hypokalaemic periodic paralysis. *Neurology* (*Minneap.*), **17,** 329.

Green, K. and Matty, A. J. (1962). Effect of thyroxine on the permeability of the isolated toad bladder. *Nature* (*Lond.*), **194,** 1190.

Griggs, R. C., Engel, W. K. and Resnick, J. S. (1970). Acetazolamide treatment of hypokalaemic periodic paralysis. Prevention of attacks and improvement of persistent weakness. *Ann. intern. Med.*, **73,** 39.

Grob, D., Johns, R. J. and Liljestrand, Ä. (1957). Potassium movement in patients with Familial Periodic Paralysis. *Amer. J. Med.*, **23,** 356.

Hamfelt, A. and Wetterberg, L. (1964). Thyrotoxic myopathy and Vitamin B6 metabolism. Report of a case with hyperthyroidism and periodic paralysis. *Acta neurol scand.*, **386.**

Hofmann, W. W. and Smith, R. A. (1970). Hypokalaemic periodic paralysis studied *in vitro*. *Brain*, **93,** 445.

Ishigami, R., Shiotani, S., Yoshida, A., Kawaya, T., Ohmoto, J., Akiyama, Y., Osawa, K., Kawaguchi, Y., Kadota, I. and Shinobe, N. (1971). Changes in serum magnesium levels in periodic paralysis (Jap.). *Jap. Arch. intern. Med.*, **18,** 17.

Itahara, K. (1961). Periodic Paralysis (Jap.). *Clin. Neurol.*, **1,** 450.

Iversen, K., Asböe-Hansen, G. and Carlsen, F. (1953). Electron microscopy of certain muscle lesions in patients with pituitary-thyroid disorders. *Acta endocr.*, **14,** 177.

Jackman, R. L. and Jones, R. E. (1964). Hyperthyroidism and periodic paralysis. *Arch. intern. Med.*, **113,** 657.

Kim, Y. T. and Cha, Y. M. (1965). *Kor. J. intern. Med.*, **8,** 237. Quoted by McFadzean and Yeung, 1967.

Kirchheiner, B. (1962). Specific muscle lesions in pituitary-thyroid disorders. *Acta med. scand.*, **172,** 539.

Lee, T. S., Kim, J. Y., Lee, J. K. and Lee, M. (1964). *J. Kor. med. Ass.*, **7,** 247. Quoted by McFadzean and Yeung, 1967.

Linder, M. A. (1955). Periodic paralysis associated with hyperthyroidism: report of three cases. *Ann. intern. Med.*, **43,** 241.

McArdle, B. (1956). Familial Periodic Paralysis. *Brit. med. Bull.*, **12,** 226.

McArdle, B. (1969). Metabolic and endocrine myopathies. In "Disorders of Voluntary Muscle". Edited by J. N. Walton, pp. 607–638. Oxford Medical Publications, London.

McFadzean, A. J. S. and Yeung, R. (1967). Periodic paralysis complicating thyrotoxicosis in Chinese. *Brit. med. J.*, **1,** 451.

Norris, F. H. Jr. (1962). Some metabolic studies of sporadic and familial periodic paralysis. *Neurology* (*Minneap.*), **12,** 208.

Norris, F. H. Jr. (1966). Status of the segmental innervation in thyrotoxic periodic paralysis. *Electroenceph. clin. Neurophysiol.*, **21,** 67.

Norris, F. H. Jr., Clark, E. C. and Biglieri, E. G. (1971). Studies in thyrotoxic periodic paralysis. *J. neurol. Sci.* (*Amst.*), **13,** 431.

Norris, F. H. Jr., Panner, B. J. and Stormont, B. M. (1968). Thyrotoxic periodic paralysis. Metabolic and ultrastructural studies. *Arch. Neurol.* (*Chic.*), **19,** 88.

Okihiro, M. M. and Beddow, R. M. (1965). Thyrotoxic periodic paralysis in Hawaii: its predilection for the Japanese race. *Neurol.* (*Minneap.*), **15,** 253.

Okinaka, S., Shizume, K., Iino, S., Watanabe, A., Irie, M., Noguchi, A., Kuma, S., Kuma, K. and Ito, T. (1957). The association of Periodic Paralysis and Hyperthyroidism in Japan. *J. clin. Endocr.*, **17,** 1454.

Overholt, E. L., Smith, V. M. and White, E. D. (1957). Periodic paralysis associated with hyperthyroidism. *Arch. intern. Med.*, **100,** 132.

Ramsay, I. D. (1965). Electromyography in thyrotoxicosis. *Quart. J. Med.*, **34,** 255.

Robertson, E. G. (1954). Thyrotoxic periodic paralysis. *Aust. Ann. Med.*, **3,** 182.

Rosenfeld, M. (1902). Acute Aufsteigende Lähmung bei Morbus Basedow. *Berl. klin. Wchnschr.*, **39,** 538.

Sagild, U. and Helweg-Larsen, H. F. (1955). Clinical picture of hereditary transistory muscular paralysis; periodic adynamia and periodic paralysis. *Nord. med.* (*Danish*), **53,** 981.

Satoyoshi, E. and Kinoshita, M. (1970). Some aspects of thyrotoxic and steroid myopathy. In "Proceedings of an International Congress on Muscle Diseases. Milan 1969". Edited by J. N. Walton, N. Canal and G. Scarlato, p. 455. Excerpta Medica, Amsterdam.

Satoyoshi, E., Murakami, K., Kowa, H., Kinoshita, M. and Nishiyama, Y. (1963a). Periodic paralysis in hyperthyroidism. *Neurology* (*Minneap.*), **13,** 746.

Satoyoshi, E., Suzuki, Y. and Abe, T. (1963b). Periodic paralysis. A study of carbohydrate and thiamine metabolism. *Neurology* (*Minneap.*), **13,** 24.

Schutta, H. S. and Armitage, J. L. (1969a). The sarcoplasmic reticulum in thyrotoxic hypokalaemic periodic paralysis. *Metabolism*, **18,** 81.

Schutta, H. S. and Armitage, J. L. (1969b). Thyrotoxic hypokalaemic periodic paralysis. *J. Neuropath. exp. Neurol.*, **28,** 321.

Seed, L. (1947). Periodic paralysis in a patient with exophthalmic goiter controlled by 6-propylthiouracil. *West. J. Surg.*, **55,** 640.

Shanes, A. M. (1958). Electrochemical aspects of physiological and pharmacological action in excitable cells. Part II. The action potential and excitation. *Pharmacol. Rev.*, **10,** 165.

Shinosaki, T. (1926). Klinische Studien über die periodische Extremitätenlähmung. *Z. ges. Neurol. Psychiat.*, **100,** 564.

Shishiba, Y., Shizume, K., Sakuma, M., Yamauchi, H., Nakao, K. and Okinaka, S. (1966). Studies on electrolyte metabolism in idiopathic and thyrotoxic periodic paralysis. III. Intra- and extracellular concentrations of potassium and sodium in muscle and their changes during induced attacks of paralysis. *Metabolism*, **15,** 153.

Shizume, K., Shishiba, Y., Sakuma, M., Yamauchi, H., Nakao, K. and Okinaka, S. (1966a). Studies on electrolyte metabolism in idiopathic and thyrotoxic periodic paralysis. I. Arterio-venous differences of electrolytes during induced paralysis. *Metabolism*, **15,** 138.

Shizume, K., Shishiba, Y., Sakuma, M., Yamauchi, H., Nakao, K. and Okinaka, S. (1966b). Studies in electrolyte metabolism in idiopathic and thyrotoxic periodic paralysis. II. Total exchangeable sodium and potassium. *Metabolism*, **15,** 145.

Shy, G. M., Wanko, T., Rowley, P. T. and Engel, A. G. (1961). Studies in Familial Periodic Paralysis. *Exp. Neurol.*, **3,** 53.

Staffurth, J. S. and Thompson, J. C. (1965). Muscle potassium in thyrotoxicosis. *Metabolism*, **14,** 241.

Talbott, J. H. (1941). Periodic paralysis: a clinical syndrome. *Medicine* (*Baltimore*), **20,** 85.

Tsuji, K. (1939). Über die Pathogenese der paroxysmalen Extremitätenlähmung. *Klin. Wchschr.*, **18,** 320.

Weber, A., Herz, R. and Reiss, I. (1963). On the mechanism of the relaxing effect of fragmented sarcoplasmic reticulum. *J. gen. Physiol.*, **46,** 679.

Winegrad, S. (1965). Autoradiographic studies of intracellular calcium in frog skeletal muscle. *J. gen. Physiol.*, **48,** 455.

Wolf, A. (1943). Effective use of thyroid in periodic paralysis. *N.Y. St. J. Med.*, **43,** 1951.

CHAPTER 4

MUSCULAR ABNORMALITIES OF HYPOTHYROIDISM

In 1880 Ord made a passing reference to the presence of muscle weakness in a woman with hypothyroidism. Since then a number of papers have been written on the subject, a confusing eponymous nomenclature has grown up, and slightly different classifications of the various muscle disorders associated with hypothyroidism have been proposed by successive authors. An attempt will be made here to give an account of the various syndromes that have been described and then to examine some of the more recent surveys of patients with hypothyroidism to see how often the syndromes are found in this disease. During the course of this review the word "hypothyroidism" refers to patients with thyroid deficiency due to primary thyroid disease; secondary hypothyroidism is used for patients with hypopituitarism. The term myxoedema is not used as it is a clinical diagnosis and only infers the presence of deposited mucopolysaccharides.

Kocher–Debré-Semelaigne syndrome

In 1892 Kocher drew attention to the presence in a young cretin of muscular enlargement, reduced power and slow movements. Thomasen (1948) reviewed several other papers in the German literature published at about the end of the nineteenth century and it is evident that their authors did not realize that there was a connection between the hypertrophic, weak muscles and the presence of cretinism. The syndrome was rediscovered by Debré and Semelaigne in 1935. Their first patient was a boy of 10 months who had hypothyroidism, arrested growth and abnormally firm hypertrophied muscles, especially of the calves. He died before treatment was started. The second patient was a girl of 2 years who had stopped growing a few months after birth; she had clear signs of hypothyroidism with retarded mental development and had pronounced generalized hypertrophy of her muscles, which were hard on palpation. Her muscle movements were slow and she was weak. She was treated with thyroid extract and within six months her muscles had become normal, all the signs of hypothyroidism had disappeared and her mental condition was nearly normal. Figure 4.1 shows the hypertrophied muscles of a hypothyroid child.

This condition has since been the subject of several reports in infants and children and is often referred to in such terms as the "infant Hercules" or "muscular athletism" (Heuyer *et al.*, 1951; Pende and Pende, 1952; Najjar and Nachman, 1965). However, the

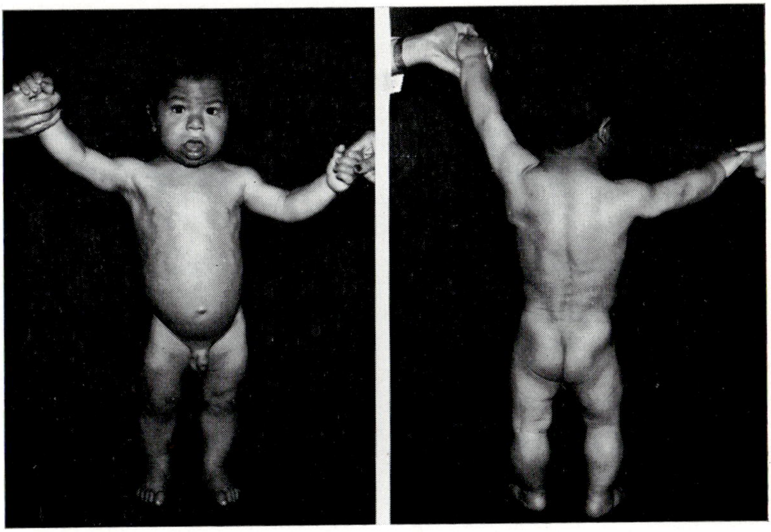

(*a*) (*b*)

Figure 4.1(*a*, *b*). Four-year-old male child with hypothyroidism showing muscular hypertrophy. (By courtesy of Dr. S. S. Najjar.)

syndrome has also been described in adults. Weitz (1931) had a male patient aged 44 in whom the condition arose when he became hypothyroid following thyroidectomy; an additional feature was the presence of diffuse muscle pains. Hesser's (1940) patient was a 30-year-old woman who developed firm, hypertrophied muscles, particularly of the calves, which gave her a rather athletic, masculine appearance. Aching and actual pain appeared in the arm and leg muscles after moderate use. It was noted that use of a particular muscle group caused further swelling of the muscle and the patient complained of a tight feeling locally. No myotonic phenomena were demonstrated. Both Weitz's and Hesser's patients were completely cured by thyroid replacement therapy and Hesser's patient relapsed when she stopped taking her medication.

Hoffman's syndrome

Shortly after Kocher's (1892) description, Hoffman (1897) found myotonoid features in a boy of 18 who had become hypothyroid after a series of partial thyroidectomies. His muscles were enlarged and firm, his movements were slow and there was delay in relaxation. After repetitive muscle use most of the difficulty in initiating movements disappeared but some stiffness and fatigue remained. Hoffmann considered that the delay in relaxation was not due to true myotonia, since even after repeated contractions of the muscle there remained a residual feeling of stiffness and tiredness. The patient was given thyroid replacement therapy, he became euthyroid and all his muscle troubles disappeared.

Since 1892 many reports have appeared in the literature (for references see Thomasen, 1948; Comings, 1962). Most, but not all, of the patients had hypertrophied muscles, slow, weak movements, painful spasms and a feeling of stiffness in the muscles on exercise, particularly in the cold. Some patients had a delay in relaxation after clenching the hand, but this improved on repetitive movement. Percussion of the muscles often produced prolonged contractions which were indistinguishable from those of myotonia. However, because of the electrical silence demonstrated by electromyography during these muscle responses, they have been referred to as "pseudomyotonia" or "myotonoid reaction" (Thomasen, 1948; Wilson and Walton, 1959).

A critical evaluation of the literature on the Kocher–Debré–Semelaigne syndrome and Hoffmann's syndrome reveals no very great points of difference. The label ascribed to any particular case seems to depend on the predominating features. For instance, Poncher and Woodward (1936) reported the case of an infant with generalized muscle hypertrophy of the Kocher–Debré–Semelaigne type who also had the myotonoid features of Hoffman's syndrome. Salick and his colleagues recently described a woman who demonstrated most of the features of both syndromes (Salick, Colachis and Pearson, 1968). An adult patient described by Norris and Panner (1966) with the features of the Kocher–Debré–Semelaigne syndrome, namely severe hypothyroidism, muscle hypertrophy and weakness, gradually developed painful muscle spasms and pseudomyotonia typical of Hoffman's syndrome as treatment with thyroxine was begun. This interesting observation raises the question as to whether or not the different manifestations of muscle disorder in hypothyroidism are related to the degree of thyroid hormone lack. Thyroid hormone deficiency appears to be greatest in athyreotic cretins and less marked in adult patients. The 2 patients described by Crispell and Parson (1954) developed myotonoid features about three or four weeks after partial thyroidectomy for thyrotoxicosis. Crispell and Parson thought that they were euthyroid, but it is now realized that sub-clinical hypothyroidism of a temporary nature is probably not uncommon after operation (Hedley *et al.*, 1971).

Muscle atrophy

Muscle atrophy in association with hypothyroidism has been described on rare occasions in the French and Italian literature; the clinical picture resembles that of muscular dystrophy (Nick, 1943; Godet-Guillain and Fardeau, 1970). However, some of the clinical observations are a little dubious and it is possible that there may have been some other underlying muscle disease (Wilson and Walton, 1959), though this is disputed (Bergouignan, Vital and Bataille, 1967).

Other muscle diseases

Myotonia congenita (Wade, 1957), myotonic dystrophy (Stanbury, Goldsmith and Gillis, 1954) and muscular dystrophy (Comings, 1962) have all been described in patients with hypothyroidism. There is no reason to believe that they are anything other than examples of a coincidental relationship. Treatment of the hypothyroidism made no difference to the symptoms of muscular dystrophy or myotonic dystrophy, though there was some improvement in Wade's (1957) patient with myotonia congenita.

The relationship between hypothyroidism and myasthenia gravis is described in Chapter 2.

Hypothyroid myopathy

It is difficult when reading the earlier accounts of muscle disorders in hypothyroidism to discover how common they are. Table 4.1 summarizes the clinical symptoms and signs referrable to the skeletal muscles from several papers published over the last 13 years. It is not suggested that they are necessarily representative of hypothyroid patients as a whole. A certain amount of selection inevitably takes place. Patients with weakness, for example, tend to present to a neurologist, patients with aches, pains and cramps to a physical

TABLE 4.1

Frequency of symptoms and signs of muscle disorder in hypothyroidism

Authors	No. of patients	Weakness %	Cramps, pains stiffness %	Hypertrophy of muscles %	Myotonoid features %
Ozker, Schumacher and Nelson (1960)	16	81	56	6	—
Aström, Kugelberg and Müller (1961)	7	70	14	0	0
Nickel *et al.* (1961)	25	28	56	0	32
Collins *et al.* (1964)	75	44	20	—	—
Totals	123	47	32	0·8	25

medicine specialist and so on; whereas patients with hypothyroidism who are seen by an endocrinologist may have minor muscle troubles overlooked because of the multiplicity of other symptoms which characterizes this disease. What is needed is a survey of an unselected series of hypothyroid patients attending all departments of a hospital, and the survey of Collings *et al.* (1964) comes nearest to this. In order to make a comparison easier, all figures in Table 4.1 have been reduced to percentages even when small numbers of patients are involved.

It can be seen that of these rather selected groups of patients, about half complained of muscle weakness and about a third had cramps, aches and pains or stiffness in their muscles. Muscle hypertrophy was very rare, being observed in only one patient out of 123 (0·8%).

An analysis of case reports (Table 4.2) gives a slightly different picture. This is not surprising, since only small numbers of highly selected patients are being described, and unusual features, such as muscular hypertrophy, tend to be emphasized. As can be seen in Table 4.2, muscular hypertrophy occurred in 27% of the cases, muscular weakness in 27% and cramps, pains and stiffness in 77%. The latter figure is probably artificially elevated by the inclusion of the patients of Golding (1970), who, as a physical medicine specialist, would tend to see hypothyroid patients presenting with muscular pain.

Weakness probably occurs in some 30 to 40% of all hypothyroid patients. It does not seem to matter what the hypothyroidism is due to, for the muscle symptoms have been noted not only in primary hypothyroidism, but also in hypothyroidism secondary to hypopituitarism (Aström, Kugelberg and Müller, 1961; Ramsay, 1971), Hashimoto's thyroiditis (David *et al.*, 1969), following radioactive iodine (Balls *et al.*, 1955; Aström, Kugelberg and Müller, 1961; Lewitus and Bornstein, 1962), thyroidectomy (Wilson and Walton, 1959; Aström, Kugelberg and Müller, 1961; Lewitus and Bornstein, 1962) and following antithyroid drugs (Thorn and Eder, 1946). The muscle weakness is usually not marked, as it may be sometimes in thyrotoxicosis, but tends to effect the same muscle groups, that is the proximal muscles of the shoulder and pelvic girdles. The movements are slow; this may be due partly to retarded cerebration and due partly to delayed contraction and relaxation of muscle (Chaney, 1924; Lambert *et al.*, 1951).

The muscles are usually of normal bulk or may rarely appear larger than normal; occasional reports have appeared of patients with muscle atrophy. When hypertrophy is present it may be localized

TABLE 4.2

Showing the main clinical features in recent cases of hypothyroid myopathy

Authors	Number of patients	Weakness	Cramps, pains or stiffness	Hypertrophy of muscles	Myotonoid features
Millikan and Haines (1953)	3	2	1	1	0
Wilson and Walton (1959)	3	0	3	1	2
Norris and Panner (1966)	1	1	0	1	0
Bergouignan *et al.* (1967)	2	1	–	0	0
Salick *et al.* (1968)	1	1	1	1	1
Pearce and Aziz (1969)	2	1	2	1	2
Hurwitz, McCormick and Allen (1970)	1	0	1	1	0
Golding (1970)	9	0	9	0	0
Totals	22	27%	77%	27%	23%

or widespread, affecting most noticeably the calves and thighs, hands, neck, tongue and facial muscles. The hypertrophied muscles usually feel firm or even indurated, though this can also apply to muscles of normal bulk. Muscle pains and stiffness frequently occur and may be present at rest, occur with exercise or be precipitated by cold weather. Painful muscle cramps, some of which simulate tetany, may be present, and opisthotonus has been noted in infants. Golding (1970) has pointed out the similarity of some of the symptoms to rheumatoid disease or polymalgia rheumatica, while Fessel (1968) believed the picture could be confused with that of polymyositis. It is worth emphasizing that many of the patients who present with muscular aches and pains, stiffness and cramps do not have obvious clinical hypothyroidism and indeed may initially have thyroid function tests which are within the normal range. It is important to repeat these thyroid function tests periodically in patients suffering from obscure muscle pains because they may later confirm the diagnosis. Possibly the tissue level of thyroid hormone is lower in these patients than their general thyroid status suggests. Routine assay of Thyroid Stimulating Hormone will probably demonstrate raised values in these patients. Wilson and Walton (1959) remarked that the symptoms could easily be dismissed as being of a psychogenic origin. One French patient from Bordeaux had made, in desperation, *diverses pérégrinations médicales en province et à Paris et qui a motivé les diagnostics les plus divers* (Bergouignan, Vital and Bataille, 1967).

The slowness of contraction and relaxation of the muscles is reflected in the characteristic delayed or "hung-up" tendon jerks, best seen in the Achilles jerk, which can be demonstrated in 80% of all hypothyroid patients (Ringqvist, 1970). This is in contrast to the virtually normal tendon jerks in patients with true myotonia. Lambert and his colleagues (1951) have shown that the cause of the prolongation of contraction and relaxation lies in the muscle itself and that nerve conduction and neuro-muscular transmission are normal; the slightly reduced body temperature of some hypothyroid patients does not account for the phenomenon. Some patients have difficulty in relaxing their muscles after a contraction, e.g. when gripping with the hand. Direct percussion of a muscle produces a "mounding phenomenon" or myoedema in about a third of hypothyroid patients (Fig. 4.2). The mounding phenomenon is painless and may last for about one minute. It is not caused by muscular contraction, for it has been shown to be electrically silent (Salick, Colachis and Pearson, 1968). It may be due to increased viscoelastic resistance.

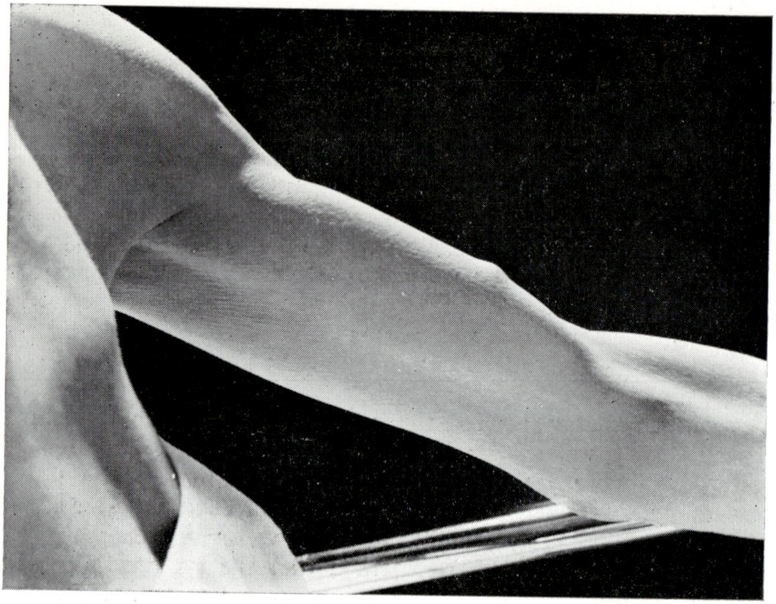

Figure 4.2. The mounding phenomenon produced by tapping the left biceps muscle of a 42-year-old female hypothyroid patient with muscular hypertrophy. (From Salick *et al.*, 1968.)

Hypothyroid neuropathy

Since limb pains, weakness of muscles and abnormal tendon reflexes could be attributed to abnormality of peripheral nerve function, the possibility of a neuropathy in hypothyroidism should be considered. Crevasse and Logue (1959) attributed the severe lancinating limb pains and paraesthesiae, which they found in 47% of 65 patients made hypothyroid by radioactive iodine, to a peripheral neuropathy, though there was little to substantiate this clinically. Nickel and Frame (1958) has also noted that subjective sensory complaints were out of proportion to objective sensory loss and they therefore exhaustively studied 25 hypothyroid patients in order to elucidate the problem further (Nickel *et al.*, 1961). All their patients complained of paraesthesiae in the fingers and toes, and of these 60% were found to have objective sensory loss in the extremities, affecting mainly pain, light touch and vibration sense. This is a much higher prevalence than has been found previously and one wonders whether it might not indicate a certain selection of cases. In a combined series reported by a Physical Medicine Department and an Endocrine Department (Ozker, Schumacher and Nelson, 1960) only 44% complained of tingling and paraesthesiae and objective signs of a neuropathy were found in a mere 12% of their patients. Reports of motor nerve conduction studies done in patients with hypothyroidism have indicated that they are normal (Lambert *et al.*, 1951; Salick, Calachis and Pearson, 1961; Norris and Panner, 1966; Fincham and Cape, 1968; Pearce and Aziz, 1969), though significant slowing of sensory nerve conduction has been demonstrated by Fincham and Cape (1968). The phenomenon of reduced conduction in the median nerve due to compression by myxoedema tissue in the carpal tunnel is, of course, well recognized (Murray and Simpson, 1958; Wayne, 1960).

Niekel and his colleagues (1961) found a basophilic metachromatic substance in a third of their patients. It was probably a mucopolysaccharide-protein complex and was infiltrating the endoneurium and perineurium of individual nerve fibres. There were also slight degenerative changes in the myelin sheaths and axis cylinders in a few patients. Pearce and Aziz (1969) found a 50% loss of myelinated fibres in the sural nerve of their patient who had evidence of segmental dymelination and remyelination.

Motor nerve conduction has been found to be abnormally low in cretins, though Moosa and Dubowitz (1971) point out that this finding is not comparable to the normal results obtained in hypothyroid adults, since the nerves of infants and young children are still undergoing myelination. They thought that the abnormally slow conduction reflected delayed maturation of the peripheral nerves.

ELECTROPHYSIOLOGICAL STUDIES

Reflex duration

In 1924 Chaney first drew attention to the use of tendon jerk reflex times in the diagnosis of primary hypothyroidism. He also showed that there was a good correlation, when the patient was treated with thyroid extract, between the patient's Basal Metabolic Rate, as it returned to normal, and the progressive shortening of the reflex time. He did not find similar changes in patients known to have low B.M.R.s for other reasons, such as pituitary tumours and anorexia nervosa.

A further report from the Mayo Clinic explored the subject in greater detail (Lambert *et al.*, 1951). Lambert and his colleagues

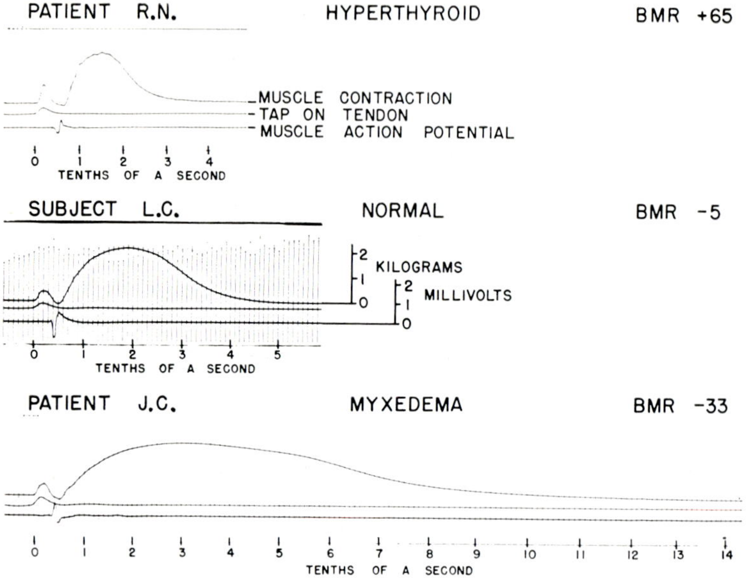

Figure 4.3. The ankle jerk in hypothyroidism (myxedema) compared to to that in normal and hyperthyroid persons. The contraction and relaxation phases are both prolonged in hypothyroidism, though the relaxation time is increased relatively more than the contraction time. (From Lambert *et al.*, 1951.)

found that measurement of the interval between the tendon hammer tap and the half relaxation time was the best measurement to make for the diagnosis of primary hypothyroidism. The contraction time and total relaxation time were both prolonged, but 45% of values for contraction time and 35% of values for relaxation time fell within the euthyroid range. Thirty-four per cent of values for total contraction and relaxation time fell within the euthyroid range. By contrast, if the tap to half relaxation time was measured, only 23% of the hypothyroid patients had a value which lay within the normal range. The values given for tap to half relaxation were (Fig. 4.3):

Normals: mean 0·34 sec. ± S.D. 0·057,
range 0·21–0·45 sec.

Hypothyroidism: mean 0·53 sec. ± S.D. 0·083,
range 0·34–0·80 sec.

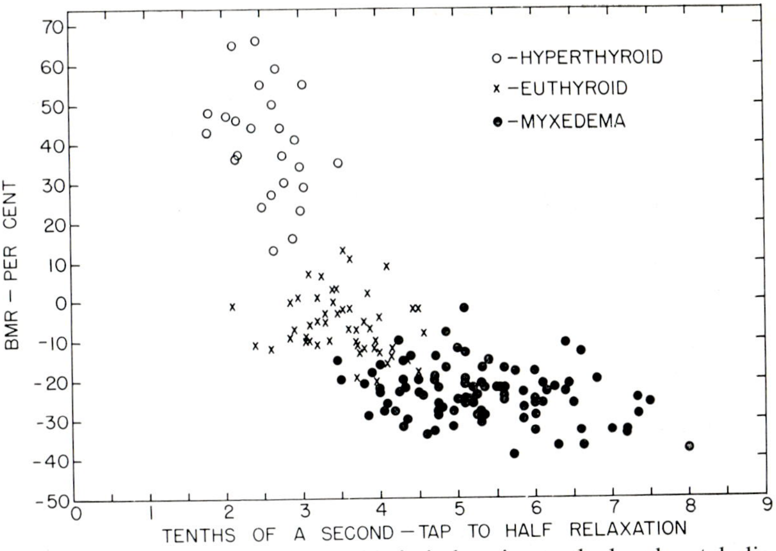

Figure 4.4. Relationship of the ankle jerk duration to the basal metabolic rate (B.M.R.) in hyperthyroid, euthyroid and hypothyroid (myxedema) patients. (From Lambert *et al.*, 1951.)

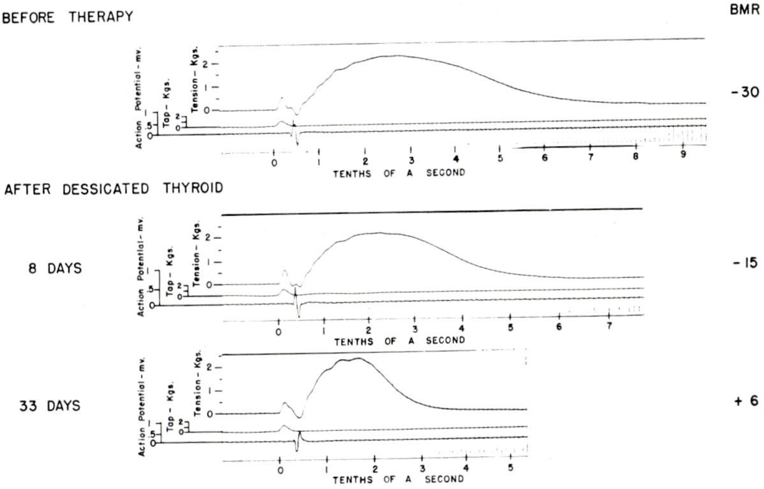

Figure 4.5. The effect of treatment with desiccated thyroid on the duration of the ankle jerk in a patient with hypothyroidism. (From Lambert *et al.*, 1951.)

The Mayo Clinic workers again showed the relationship of the B.M.R. to the duration of the ankle jerk (Fig. 4.4) and demonstrated the return of the jerk towards normal as the patient was given thyroid hormone replacement (Fig. 4.5).

They showed that the slow relaxation was not due to delayed nerve conduction, for the interval of tap to the beginning of contraction was the same in hypothyroid patients as in controls, and they confirmed this by nerve conduction studies. They also demonstrated electromyographically that the slow relaxation was not due to a tetanic type of stimulation or to myotonia. Although there was a slight difference in mean temperature between the muscle of normal and hypothyroid subjects, this was not sufficient to account for the difference in the duration of the ankle jerk. They concluded that "the slow response must be caused by an abnormality of the muscle itself, either an increase in viscosity due to the myxoedematous infiltration of the muscle as suggested by Harrell and Daniel (1941) or a decrease in the rate of energy liberation in the contractile process".

Subsequent experience with the measurement of ankle jerk duration has largely confirmed its value in the assessment of thyroid function (Lawson, 1958; Bowers, Gordon and Segaloff, 1959; Sharpe, 1961; Mann, 1963; Ekbom *et al.*, 1966; Ringqvist, 1970). However, too much emphasis should not be placed on it as a diagnostic test. It is only about 80% accurate in the diagnosis of hypothyroidism (Ringqvist, 1970) and its true value lies in the assessment of the results of treatment, since the test has a high degree of reproducibility in the individual patient (Kissel, Hartemann and Duc, 1965). It should be remembered that a prolonged duration time does not only occur in primary hypothyroidism. It has been observed in hypothermia, oedema of the leg, diabetes, parkinsonism, neurosyphilis, sarcoidosis, sprue and pernicious anaemia (Waal-Manning, 1969). Drugs such as procaine amide, quinidine, reserpine and propranolol were also found to prolong the duration of the Achilles tendon reflex (Waal-Manning, 1969). It is obviously important to be aware of these extraneous factors when interpreting reflex durations in patients with thyroid disease. Moreover, Weissbein and Lawson (1960) have actually observed an increase in muscle contraction time in hypothyroid patients given small doses of replacement therapy.

Electromyography

Reports about a variety of electromyographic changes occurring

TABLE 4.3

Electromyographic findings in hypothyroidism

Authors	No. of patients	Reduction in action potential duration	Reduction in amplitude	Increase in polyphasics	Insertional activity or hyper-irritability	Fibrillation	Fasciculation	Positive sharp waves	Repetitive chains of discharges after reflex motion	Action potentials during cramp	Electrical silence of myoedema
Pipberger, Kälin and Wegmann (1955)	5	3	3	3					1		
Ross *et al.* (1958)	1	0			1	0	0				
Waldstein *et al.* (1958)	20*	7	7	14	14				15		
Wilson and Walton (1959)	2	0	0	0	0	0	0		0		
Ozker, Schumacher and Nelson (1960)	16				11	8	4	2	4		
Aström, Kugelberg and Müller (1961)	8	7	7	7	0	0	0	0			
Nickel *et al.* (1961)	5	†	5								
Norris and Panner (1966)	1	1	1	0	0						
Bergouignan, Vital and Bataille (1967)	2	1	0	2							
Fessel (1968)	2	0	0	0	0	0	0	0	0		
Salick, Colachis and Pearson (1968)	1	1		1	1	1		1	1		1
Hurwitz, McCormick and Allen (1970)	1									1	
	64%	31%	36%	42%	42%	14%	6%	5%	32%	2%	2%

* Consecutive. † Reduced number of motor discharges.

in hypothyroidism have appeared in the last 12 years or so (Table 4.3). Different investigators have used different methods, such as external electrodes, external and intramuscular electrodes and bipolar intramuscular electrodes, so that it is difficult to know if one is comparing like with like. However, Table 4.3 summarizes the positive findings which have been recorded by various workers. Where there is a blank in a column, it means that the authors have not said whether or not they have looked for a particular phenomenon. Thus, although the analysis of the frequency with which different abnormalities may be found in hypothyroidism is not entirely accurate, it will nevertheless give some sort of guide.

Insertional activity and hyperirritability were found in 42% of the patients and was one of the commonest abnormalities. Waldstein *et al.* (1958) pointed out that, in normal subjects, movement of an electrode in muscle evokes a very short burst of electrical activity, whereas in the hypothyroid patients there was often a sequence of irregular, high voltage potentials which lasted three to five times as long as normal. Exactly the same thing was noted after percussion of the muscle with a tendon hammer. The hyperirritability tended to disappear following treatment with thyroid hormones (Waldstein *et al.*, 1958; Ross *et al.*, 1958). In addition, 32% of the patients showed repetitive chains of potentials after tapping the muscle tendon. These phenomena are all rather similar to those which occur in both myotonia congenita (Thomsen's disease) and dystrophia myotonica. However, none of the "dive bomber" sounds produced by the decrescendo frequency of the repetitive discharges of true myotonia have been found in hypothyroidism apart from a suggestion of it in one patient (Salick, Colachis and Pearson, 1968). Nevertheless, Lambert and Sayre (1955) found trains of positive spikes and waves, similar to the electrical activity of myotonic muscle, in rabbits following thyroidectomy. The abnormalities disappeared three to six weeks after the rabbits had been put on thyroid replacement therapy. Earlier, Lambert and his colleagues (1951) had found some repetitive discharges in patients with hypothyroidism following the elicitation of the tendon jerk. They concluded that there was no true myotonia in hypothyroidism because the duration of the ankle jerk is shorter than normal in myotonia, rather than longer as in hypothyroidism, and that repetitive after-discharges were not constantly present and related to the length of the ankle jerk duration. It seems unlikely that repetitive firing off of motor units is the cause of the prolonged muscular contraction of hypothyroidism. However, a significant proportion of patients do show mechanical irritability of muscle fibres which may fire off randomly and perhaps even be associated with cramps (Hurwitz, McCormick and Allen, 1970).

Polyphasic potentials occurred in 42% of the patients studied electromyographically. In some, up to 50% of the potentials were of this type (Waldstein *et al.*, 1958). This, of course, may be found in either myopathies or neuropathies, but the presence of a reduced mean action potential duration in 31% of patients would tend to suggest that the abnormality in hypothyroidism lay in muscle rather than nerve, since in neurogenic paresis the action potential duration is either normal or increased (Buchthal, 1957), while in myopathies it is decreased (Kugelberg, 1947, 1949; Buchthal and Rosenfalck, 1963). In 2 patients with muscular hypertrophy as the sole abnormality, Pipberger, Kälin and Wegman (1955) found an increase in the duration of motor unit potentials. This has not been found by others since.

It is rather more difficult to be sure what the reported incidence of fibrillation (14%), fasciculation (6%) and positive sharp waves (5%) mean. Normally they imply denervation and fasciculation usually denotes anterior horn cell disease. However, single action potentials of short duration which are virtually identical to fibrillation potentials may be found in myotonia and in the end-plate region of normal muscle and "benign" fasciculations are sometimes observed which do not denote anterior horn cell disease. Moreover, in severe myopathies, short potentials, which are indistinguishable from denervation potentials, may occasionally be seen. It is thus almost impossible to comment on the significance of these phenomena, and their presence should probably be ignored in trying to decide the site of the lesion in hypothyroidism. On the whole, the evidence favours a myopathy in that three major criteria for the diagnosis of a myopathy have been described—namely, reduction in action potential duration, reduction in amplitude and an increase in polyphasics. The fibrillation potentials are not incompatible with a myopathy, though it is conceivable that the denervation potentials could mean that there is some involvement of terminal nerve fibres with denervation of individual fibres (Pearce and Aziz, 1969). Repetitive chains of discharges following reflex movement might represent a myotonia-like phenomenon or could be insertional activity caused by mechanical movement of the needle as a result of muscle contraction. In this context, it is of interest to note that three of the papers which describe it in hypothyroid patients also record a high incidence of insertional activity (see Table 4.3,

Waldstein *et al.*, 1958; Ozker, Schumacher and Nelson, 1960; Salick, Colachis and Pearson, 1968).

No real difference in the electromyographic findings can be defined between those patients presenting with hypertrophic muscles and those with normal muscle bulk. Both have evidence of reduced action potential duration, an increase in polyphasics, insertional activity and chains of repetitive discharges after reflex motion. However, there may be a spectrum of E.M.G. changes in hypothyroidism, possibly dependent on the degree of thyroid hormonal deficiency, for Norris and Panner's (1966) patient who presented with hypertrophied muscles did not develop excessive polyphasics on the E.M.G. until treatment had been given, his muscles had returned to normal bulk and he was beginning to experience muscle spasms. The patient had noted that he had had the same muscle spasms much earlier on in his illness but they had disappeared as the weakness progressed.

The "mounding phenomenon", previously referred to, which consists of a ridge of muscle that results from the muscle being tapped with a reflex hammer, is electrically silent (Norris and Panner, 1966; Salick and Pearson, 1967; Pearce and Aziz, 1969), so it cannot be due to contraction of muscle fibres but must reflect a temporary alteration of the physiochemical structure of the muscle fibres.

Although the existence of a neuropathy in hypothyroidism has been suggested by Crevasse and Logue (1959) and by Nickel and his colleagues (1961), there is little electrophysiological evidence to support this. Motor nerve conduction times have been reported within the normal range (Lambert *et al.*, 1951; Norris and Panner, 1966; Salick, Colachis and Pearson, 1968; Pearce and Aziz, 1969), though of course the phenomenon of compression of the median nerve in the carpal tunnel is well recognized in hypothyroid patients with myxoedema (Murray and Simpson, 1958; Wayne, 1960). Whether sensory neuropathy really occurs in hypothyroidism is not yet known as in only one study has slowing of sensory nerve conduction been demonstrated (Fincham and Cape, 1968).

Norris and Panner (1966) thought that their patient had some evidence of a defect in transmission across the motor end-plate. Edrophonium made no difference to the muscle weakness while the patient was hypothyroid. Electromyographic studies were not carried out until two weeks after he had been placed on thyroxine. The E.M.G. findings were not similar to those of myasthenia gravis, that is to say there was not a progressive decrease in amplitude following repetition nerve stimulation, but there was some improvement in amplitude following 10 mg of edrophonium intravenously and direct stimulation of the muscle fibres resulted in potentials which were maintained normally. Clearly more work needs to be done on the behaviour of the motor end-plate in hypothyroidism.

Biochemistry

Very little is known about the biochemical changes which take place in muscle in hypothyroidism and comprehensive information is only available in humans about creatine and creatinine excretion and serum levels of creatine phosphokinase (CPK, adenosine 5′-triphosphate-creatine phosphotransferase).

Creatine and creatinine

Thyroid insufficiency is nearly always associated with the absence of creatinuria (Shorr, Richardson and Wolff, 1933; Poncher, Visscher and Woodward, 1934) and a normal excretion of creatinine (Kuhlbäck, 1957). There is an increased tolerance to ingested creatine in hypothyroidism (Thorn, 1936). In 7 patients Thorn (1936) found a retention of between 86 and 95% of ingested creatine, unlike the situation in hyperthyroidism where creatine tolerance is markedly diminished (see p. 18). After his patients were started on thyroid replacement therapy tolerance to administered creatine fell. This was most noticeable early in the course of treatment. At the same time creatinuria developed within 48 hours of the commencement of therapy with 100–200 mg of thyroid extract (equals 0·15–0·3 mg L-thyroxine approx.), and reached its maximum of 300–600 mg per 24 hours at seven days. These changes in creatine excretion preceded a rise in the basal metabolic rate, weight loss or clinical signs of improvement. Later on, when the thyroid replacement therapy had been given for a longer period and the basal metabolic rate had become normal the creatinuria diminished and the tolerance to ingested creatine improved.

Creatine phosphokinase

The enzyme creatine phosphokinase which catalyses the reversible transference of a phosphoryl group from creatine phosphate to adenosine diphosphate in order to form adenosine triphosphate (creatine phosphate + ADP $\rightleftharpoons$ creatine + ATP) has been found by many authors to be elevated (Table 4.4). In the two more recent series of Graig and Smith (1965) and of Griffiths (1965) round about

90% of patients had elevated serum CPK levels. Graig and Smith (1965) measured CPK levels in patients with hyper-, eu- and hypothyroidism and showed that there was a good inverse correlation between PBI values and serum CPK levels (Fig. 4.6). Follow-up studies done on individual patients showed a decline in CPK values to normal levels as they were rendered euthyroid with thyroid replacement therapy. Griffiths (1965) found that in most of the patients the levels came down to normal within a month of the start of treatment and all of them had normal values by the time they were thought to be clinically euthyroid. In fact, it seems possible that, in patients with an initially raised CPK, serial enzyme levels

TABLE 4.4

Prevalence of elevated serum creatine phosphokinase levels in hypothyroidism

Authors	No. of patients	% with elevated serum CPK levels
Graig and Ross (1963)	15	66
Saito *et al.* (1963)	8*	100
Hess *et al.* (1964)	5	20
Graig and Smith (1965)	30	87
Griffiths (1965)	39	90
Ekbom *et al.* (1966)	6	100

* Seven were cretins.

may be of help in establishing the correct dose of replacement thyroxine. Certainly, Ekbom and his colleagues (1966) felt that it gave a better indication of thyroid status than ankle jerk duration measurements.

It is difficult to link the raised serum CPK levels with the absence of creatinuria in these patients, for in muscular dystrophy of the Duchenne type there is a similar rise in CPK but there is also an increase in creatinuria, while in hyperthyroidism the creatinuria is associated with lowered levels of CPK. It has been suggested (Graig and Smith, 1965) that CPK leaks out of muscle in hypothyroid patients. However, Griffiths (1965) thought that heart muscle was a more likely source of CPK than skeletal muscle, because he found that the patterns of CPK in hypothyroidism and myocardial

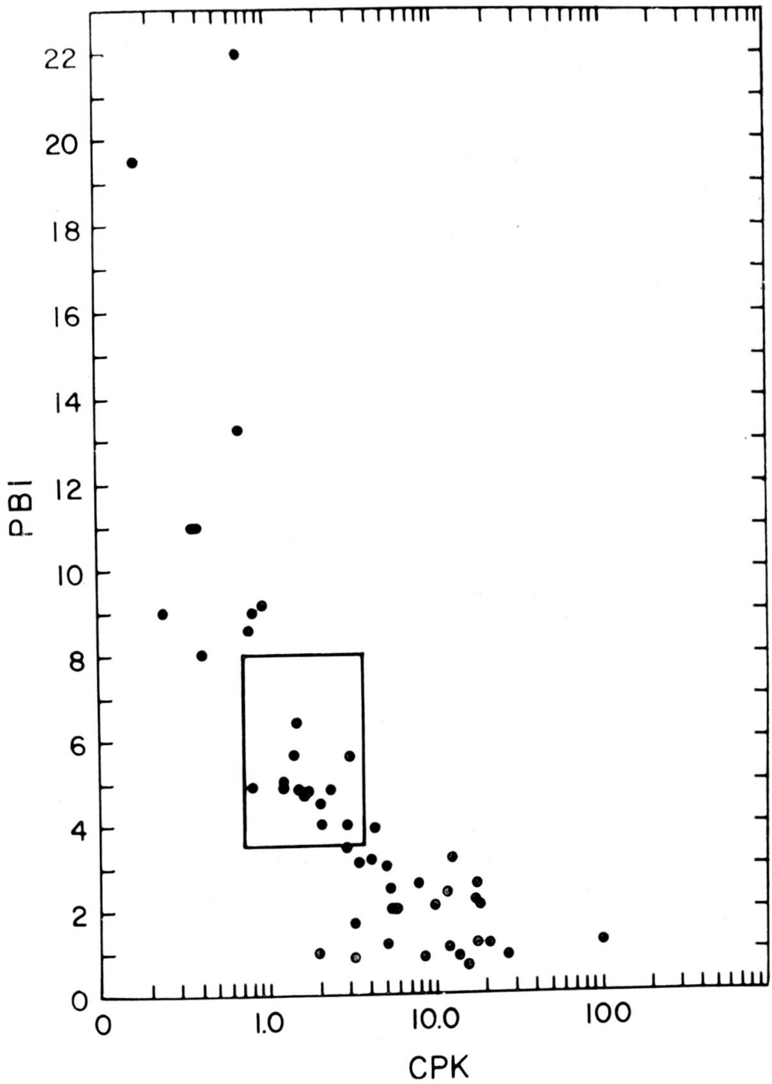

Figure 4.6. Correlation between serum CPK (units) and the PBI (μg/100 ml). The enclosed area indicates the ranges of normality. (From Graig and Smith, 1965.)

infarction were remarkably similar and differed quite a lot from that seen in muscular dystrophy. Obviously more work on the isoenzymes of CPK using starch gel electrophoresis (Sjövall and Voigt, 1964) needs to be done in order to resolve the problem.

Other muscle enzymes

There is less information about other enzymes, but raised levels of serum glutamic oxaloacetic transaminase, glutamic pyruvate transaminase, lactic dehydrogenase, aldolase and malic dehydrogenase have all been reported in some patients with hypothyroidism (Lieberthal, Benson and Klitgaard, 1963; Griffiths, 1965; Graig and Smith, 1965; Pearce and Aziz, 1969; Hurwitz, McCormick and Allen, 1970). Studies on muscle enzymes in biopsy tissue have been scanty. Fessel (1968) found a decrease in phosphorylase in the 2 patients he biopsied, but Hurwitz and his colleagues (1970) found a normal phosphorylase along with succinic dehydrogenase, lactic dehydrogenase, malate dehydrogenase, creatine phosphokinase, aldolase, amylo-1, 6-glucosidase and phosphofrucktokinase. Muscle glycogen content was normal. One muscle enzyme, α-glucosidase (lysosomal acid-maltase), was found to be abnormally low by Hurwitz, McCormick and Allen (1970) in three separate muscle biopsies taken from their patient before treatment. The level rose to the low-normal range six months after the start of L-thyroxine therapy. The authors commented that it was difficult to explain the association of a low α-glucosidase level and a normal concentration of glycogen in the muscle. Although low α-glucosidase levels have been found in the muscles of 2 further patients with hypothyroid myopathy (Engel and Gomez, 1970), work on hypothyroid rats has failed to show any reduction in α-glucosidase (acid maltase) activity in muscle (Koster, 1970; McCormick, Allen and Hurwitz, 1971). It is possible that the deficiency of this enzyme was not caused primarily by hypothyroidism in the case of Hurwitz, McCormick and Allen (1970), but that the low levels of the enzyme may have contributed to the weakness. Engel (1970) has described acid maltase deficiency in adults with a myopathy but with no evidence of hypothyroidism.

Norris and Panner (1966) studied histochemically a biopsy from a patient with hypothyroid myopathy and found normal amounts of diphosphopyridine nucleotide dehydrogenase, diphosphopyridine-linked lactate dehydrogenase, succinate dehydrogenase, cytochrome oxidase, diphosphopyridine-linked α-glycerophosphate dehydrogenase, menadione-linked α-glycerophosphate dehydrogenase, phosphorylase, A-band adenosine triphosphatase, glycogen and uridine diphosphate glucose-glycogen transferase.

Magnesium

Although Kleeman and his colleagues (1958) found no difference in serum magnesium between hypothyroid and normal subjects, Kobayashi and Takeuchi (1967) claimed that hypothyroid patients tended to have high levels. However, they did not provide any statistical evidence and the numbers studied were small.

Sodium and potassium

Aikawa (1956) found that the serum sodium tended to be low in hypothyroid patients and that the exchangeable sodium was increased. With thyroid replacement therapy the serum sodium rose and the exchangeable sodium fell. There was little alteration in the values for exchangeable potassium. These results have been largely confirmed by Munro, Renschler and Wilson (1958). Aikawa (1956) thought that the sodium changes were produced by the osmotic effect of the hyaluronic acid deposited in the extravascular, extracellular compartment. This would lead to an increase in the interstitial fluid volume, an increase in total body sodium and a concomitant fall in circulating blood volume and serum sodium.

Arons and his colleagues (1956) found low exchangeable potassium values in 5 out of 9 hypothyroid patients and normal exchangeable sodium values in 8. No consistent changes in exchangeable sodium or Na^e/K^e ratios were found after treatment. However, studies of total body electrolytes are difficult and the range of normal values is wide (Edelman *et al.*, 1952). In the absence of strong corroborative evidence from different centres, it is probable that changes in sodium and potassium cannot be interpreted with reference to the myopathy of hypothyroidism. The difficulty in these studies is the masking hydrophilic effect of the myxoedema tissue.

Pathology

Light microscopy. Light microscopy has shown abnormalities in almost all muscle biopsy tissue taken from patients with hypothyroidism, though the changes have been disregarded by some authors (Adams, Denny-Brown and Pearson, 1962; Adams, 1969). As can be seen in Table 4.5 the most common appearance was one of degeneration which occurred in 61% of the patients and which was usually confined to small numbers of fibres scattered at random

TABLE 4.5

*Showing the relative frequency of histological changes on light microscopy of muscle from 33 patients with hypothyroidism**

		%
No. of patients	33	100
Focal necrosis	20	61
Focal basophilia of fibres	14	42
Vacuolization of fibres	5	15
Variation in fibre size	5	15
Mucoproteins demonstrated	11	33
Increase in sarcolemmal nuclei	15	45
Central positioning of nuclei	13	39
Perinuclear haloes	1	3
Presence of hyperplastic nuclei	9	27
Lymphocytic infiltration	6	18
Fat in connective tissue	2	6

* Hesser (1940); Foster and Barr (1944); Thomasen (1948); Brewer (1951); Berkheiser (1955); Marshall and McCaughey (1956); Ross *et al.* (1958); Wilson and Walton (1959); Aström, Kugelberg and Müller (1961); Nickel *et al.* (1961); Norris and Panner (1966); Bergouignan, Vital and Bataille (1967); Fessel (1968); Salick, Colachis and Pearson (1968); Hurwitz, McCormick and Allen (1970).

through the muscle. Segments of the muscle fibres showed hyalinization and granular and vacuolar degeneration (Aström, Kugelberg and Müller, 1961). The larger fibres measuring 90 to 100 μ in diameter tended to show structural changes, consisting of cloudiness and a granular appearance of the cytoplasm, and loss of striations and myofibrils (Nickel *et al.*, 1961). Sometimes the muscle fibres were noted to be very variable in size. Large and small fibres were seen alongside each other in a haphazard way. Aström, Kugelberg and Müller (1961) commented on the small size of the muscle fibres in their patients, mostly under 50 μ in diameter, occasionally as small as 15 μ or less and found very few large fibres of 100 μ or more. On the other hand, Hurwitz, McCormick and Allen (1970) found the mean diameter of their patient's muscle fibres to be 84 μ compared with a mean figure for controls of 45 μ. However, it is the variability in size which has impressed most authors who have commented about the morphology of the muscle fibres. For instance, in the patient of Salick, Colachis and Pearson (1968) they varied from 20 to 115 μ; also, instead of the usual polygonal shape on cross section, the fibres tended to be rounded.

Cheek and his colleagues (1966) found that the individual cell mass of cretins was reduced whether on an age or body size basis. The number of muscle fibres appeared to be normal, but their protein content was reduced. After 11 months of thyroid therapy the muscle fibre size of two cretinous twins showed a definite increase, while the fibre population remained the same. Cheek *et al.* (1966) compared these findings with those in older children with acquired hypothyroidism. Four out of the 7 showed enlarged muscle fibres when related to body size and in all 7 there was a decrease in size when thyroid therapy was given. Moreover, in 6 of them there was an increase in the number of fibres. The reasons for the differences between the two groups was not entirely clear but may have been related to the severe degree of hypothyroidism in the cretins with a consequent great reduction in the synthesis of cell protein (Tata *et al.*, 1963).

Spiro and his co-workers (1970) have recently described the characteristics of the muscle fibres in a cretin aged 3½ years and in a cretinous baby aged 2 months. Whereas the latter showed no abnormalities of any sort compared with normal controls matched for age, the former, who had "hypertrophied" muscles, showed several abnormalities. There was atrophy, predominantly of Type I fibres, abnormalities of oxidative enzymatic activity, focal collections of glycogen in the subsarcolemmal area and distension of the sarcoplasmic reticulum. After treatment the muscle hypertrophy disappeared and the muscle became microscopically and histochemically normal.

Just under half of the hypothyroid muscles examined (Table 4.5) showed some abnormality of the nuclei. In 45% there was an increase in the number of sarcolemmal nuclei. In 39% nuclei were found in the centre of the fibre rather than immediately underneath the sarcolemma, which is their normal position, and in 27% the nuclei were noted to be hyperplastic. These nuclear changes, plus the basophilic staining of the muscle sarcoplasm seen in 42% of the patients, suggest that some regeneration of muscle was taking place. Other histological changes which have been infrequently found are lymphocytic infiltration and the presence of fat in the connective tissue. In a patient with hypertrophied muscles Pearce and Aziz (1969) noted marked vacuolation of the larger fibres. The vacuoles were mainly centrally placed in the myofibrils.

It is not entirely clear whether myxoedema tissue infiltrates the skeletal muscles. Watson and Pearce (1947) found that this mucinous material was composed of two acid polysaccharides, chondroitin sulphuric acid and hyaluronic acid, combined in some way with protein. The material stains metachromatically and has been clearly demonstrated in the skin and connective tissue of patients with primary hypothyroidism. Similar material has been found in the musculature of the tongue and Foster and Barr (1944) suggested that the widespread infiltrations found at autopsy in the cardiac, skeletal and smooth muscles of their patient were composed of mucoid. Similar infiltrations, thought to be composed of a mucopolysaccharide, have been found in the sternomastoid (Berkheiser, 1955), in the tongue and in the myocardium (Brewer, 1951).

Asböe-Hansen, Iversen and Wichmann (1952) found semilunar or crescent shaped subsarcolemmal deposits on cross section, which were spindle-shaped when seen in longitudinal section, in one out of 7 patients with myxoedema. Kirchheiner (1962) reported similar lesions in six out of 10 muscle biopsies in patients with myxoedema. These findings have also been described by Spiro *et al.* (1970) in a cretinous child. Asböe-Hansen and his colleagues (1952) found that this material consisted of acid mucopolysaccharides.

Bergouignan and his colleagues (1967) found ringed fibres in their two patients. These may occur in normal muscle, particularly in gastrocnemius and are frequently seen in muscular dystrophies and in myotonic dystrophy (Bethlem and Wijngaarden, 1963). Lapresle and Fardeau (1965) found annular fibres in 5 cases out of 13 with hypothyroid myopathy. It is difficult to know how significant they are in hypothyroidism, but it is conceivable that they could have some relationship to the peculiar mechanical properties of the muscles of these patients.

In summary, then, the major changes which take place in the skeletal muscles of hypothyroid patients are areas of focal necrosis of muscle fibres, great variability in the size of the muscle fibres and evidence of regeneration, as evidenced by the increase in size and number of sarcolemmal nuclei and their central position. It is interesting to compare these findings in humans with the histological changes described by Lambert and Sayre (1955) in rabbits which had been thyroidectomized four to eight weeks previously. "Histologic examination of biopsy specimens revealed vacuolated muscle fibres, fibres in various stages of hyaline degeneration and some evidence of regeneration. Degenerative changes appeared first in the sacro-spinalis muscle, but involved thigh, thoracic spinal, shoulder girdle and other muscles as the condition became more severe." Lambert and Sayre found that if the rabbits were allowed to remain hypothyroid for a period of many months the abnormalities diminished gradually but never entirely disappeared. As time went on muscle fibres were gradually replaced by fat cells. In all their histological material the nerve fibres appeared normal. The changes they described seemed to be closely related to the hypothyroid state, for of the 29 rabbits operated upon, 23 developed degenerative changes in muscle, while the 6 rabbits without changes were found to have had incomplete thyroidectomies. Out of 38 control rabbits, one showed moderate degenerative lesions, 5 showed minimal changes and 32 showed no abnormality. In 5 thyroidectomized rabbits treatment with triiodothyronine gradually restored the structure of the muscle fibres and degenerative lesions appeared once again when the replacement therapy was stopped.

Electron microscopy. Electron microscopy studies of muscle in hypothyroidism are extremely limited, only 5 patients having been examined in this way (Norris and Panner, 1966; Bergouignan, Vital and Bataille, 1967; Godet-Guillain and Fardeau, 1970; Hurwitz, McCormick and Allen, 1970). Hurwitz and his colleagues (1970) found generalized sarcolemmal thickening and focal myofibrillar degeneration. Norris and Panner (1966) were unable to find any changes in the sarcolemma or in the sarcoplasmic reticulum of their case. There were, however, small, scattered areas of ultrastructural change. These consisted of areas with increased numbers of sarcolemmal nuclei or areas in which there had been central migration of nuclei. Nucleoli were prominent in many of the nuclei. Myofilaments were absent and round many of the subsarcolemmal nuclei were clumps of mitochondria and lipofuscin granules. They examined the areas of muscle which had been shown to exhibit sarcoplasmic basophilia on light microscopy and found that they represented localized segments of total structural disorganization. There was no orderly arrangement of myofilaments, just fibrillar debris. There was no evidence of muscle regeneration and, although sarcoplasmic basophilia has been considered to indicate an increased ribonucleic acid content, which accompanies muscle regeneration (Adams, Denny-Brown and Pearson, 1962), Norris and Panner were unable to find either increased numbers of ribosomes or immature myofilaments in these areas. In other areas there was an irregular loss of myofilaments (Fig. 4.7), with replacement by glycogen in some instances (Fig. 4.8). It was not thought that the glycogen infiltration was responsible for the disorganization and loss of myofilaments, since this occurred whether or not glycogen was present in the area. In areas of focal myofibrillar change Godet-Guillain and Fardeau (1970) found either dilatation or proliferation of the sarcoplasmic reticulum into tubular "complexes".

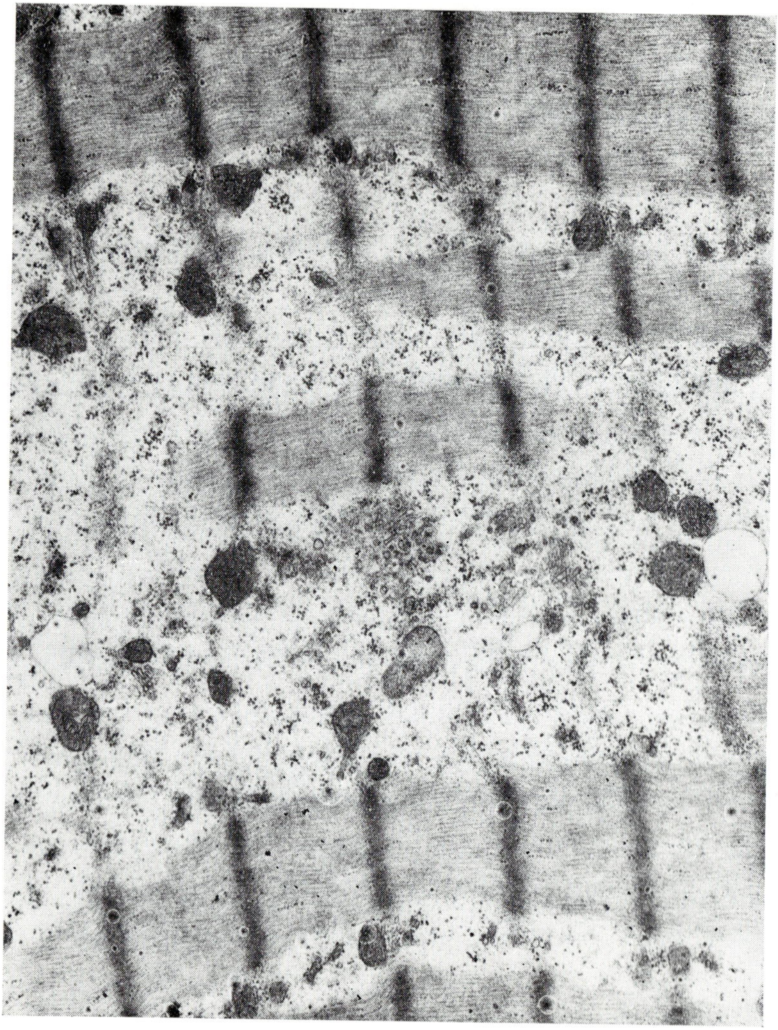

Figure 4.7. Foci of fibre degeneration. There is interruption of the myofibrils and an increased distance between them. The Z bands can still be faintly seen. There are normal glycogen granules and a few vesicles (×15,700). (From Norris and Panner, 1966.)

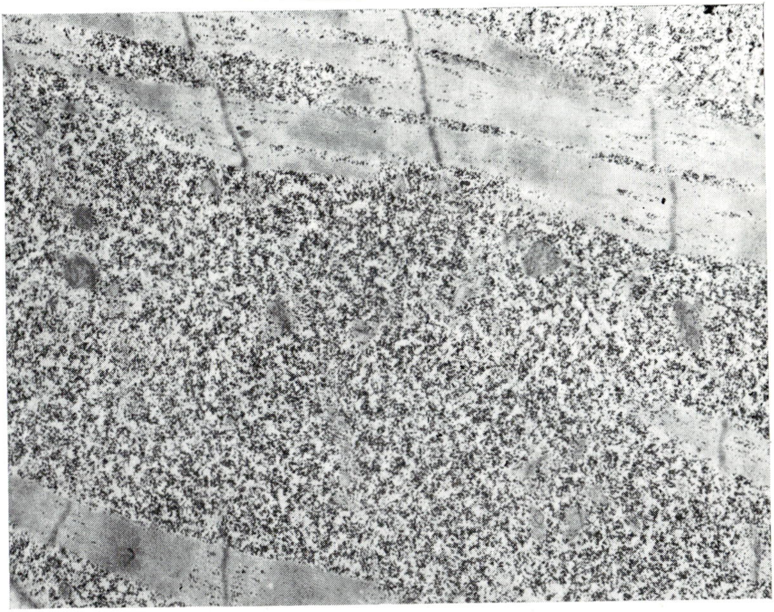

Figure 4.8. Irregular fragmentation of myofibrils and increased glycogen deposition (×16,500). (From Norris and Panner, 1966.)

Norris and Panner (1966) also noted changes in a small number of mitochondria. These consisted either of dense, round inclusion bodies which resembled lipid (Fig. 4.9) or of unusual rearrangements of mitochondrial cristae into box-like forms or linear and para-crystalline forms (Fig. 4.10). These abnormal mitochondrial configurations were found most commonly in the mitochondrial clusters round nuclei but were also present in deeper interfibrillar regions. There was no correlation between the areas having such mitochondria and the areas showing loss of myofilaments.

Godet-Guillain and Fardeau (1970) found a high incidence of mitochondrial structural change. Rectangular bodies were formed inside the cristae, composed of four parallel sheets joined transversely (Fig. 4.11). Other mitochondrial inclusions were more amorphous. It is difficult to be certain what the mitochondrial changes mean, for somewhat similar arrangements of cristae have been found by Luft *et al.* (1962) in a case of non-thyroidal hypermetabolism and by Gustaffson and his colleagues (1965) in both hypo- and hyper-thyroid rats.

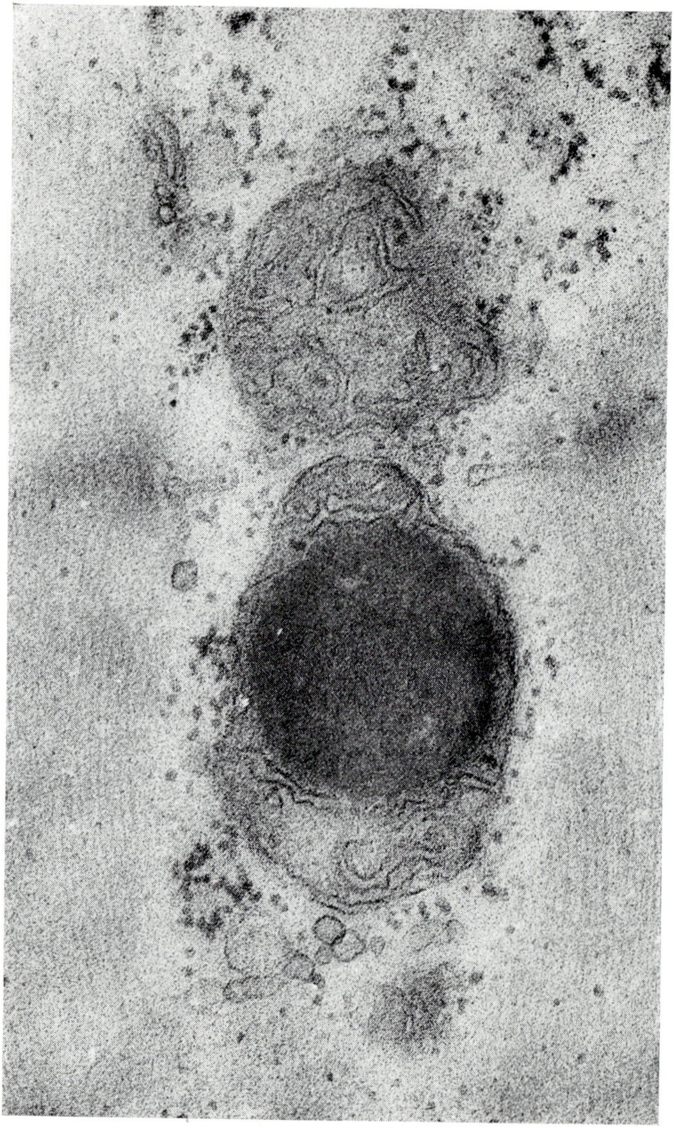

Figure 4.9. Mitochondrion containing a large dense body (× 37,000). (From Norris and Panner, 1966.)

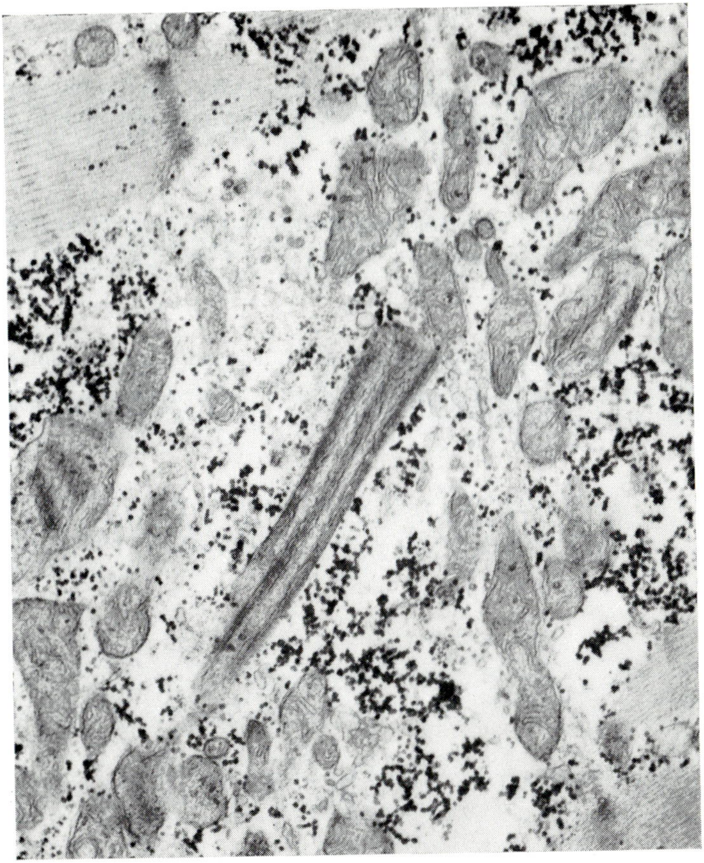

Figure 4.10. Linear and paracrystalline cristal configurations are seen in the mitochondrion in the centre of the picture. Other mitochondria show lesser degrees of change (×17,000). (From Norris and Panner, 1966.)

The lipofusion granules found by Norris and Panner (1966) were present in greatest numbers beneath the sarcolemma and round nuclei, though a few were deeper in the muscle fibres. The appearance of the granules was variable. Frequently there was an almost complete limiting membrane and they contained short fibrils of unknown origin, dense granules and lipid droplets (Fig. 4.12). Since Norris and Panner found similar structures within the cytoplasm of inter-

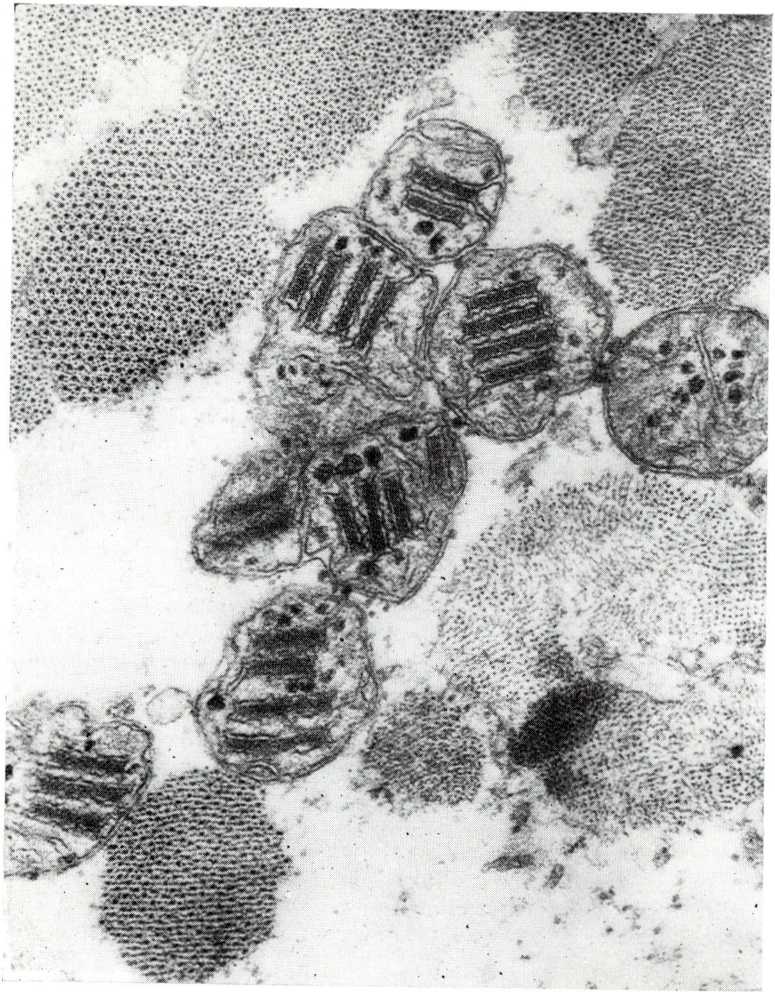

Figure 4.11. Deltoid muscle of a 63-year-old woman with hypothyroid myopathy. Specimen fixed in osmium tetroxide 2% at 0°C for 2 hours 30 min. and stained with uranyl acetate and lead citrate. Within the mitochondrial cristae are seen rectangular inclusions which are formed by transversely arranged parallel striations. (From Godet-Guillain and Fardeau, 1970.)

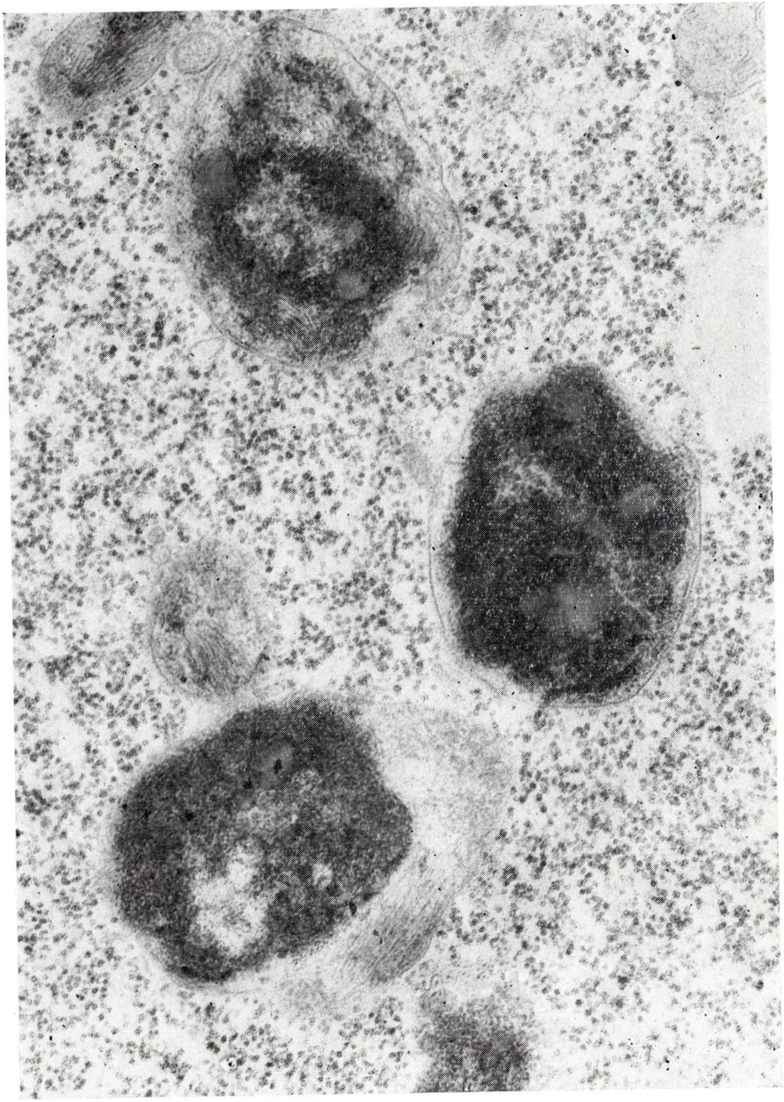

Figure 4.12. Dense lipofuscin bodies containing variable proportions of short fibrils, granules and lipid droplets (×16,000). (From Norris and Panner, 1966.)

stitial cytoplasm they suggested that some of the lipofuscin granules must get extruded from muscle cells.

Norris and Panner (1966) found none of the "half-moons" described in one case of myxoedema by Asböe-Hansen and his colleagues (1952).

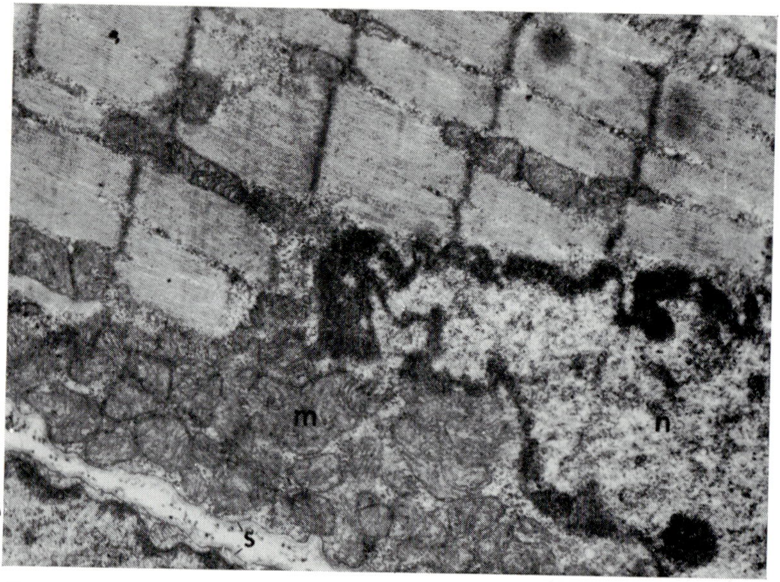

Figure 4.13. Electron micrograph showing portions of two adjacent leg muscle fibres from a hypothyroid rat. There are a large number of mitochondria (M) in the sarcoplasm adjacent to the nucleus (N). The mitochondrial matrix is denser than normal and the cristae are more closely packed. The border of the fibres is marked by S. (× 18,000). Compare with Fig. 4.14(b). (From Gustafsson *et al.*, 1965.)

In their electron microscopic study of 2 patients Bergouignan and his colleagues (1967) noted the abundance of annular myofibrils already referred to in the section on light microscopy. They did note, like Norris and Panner (1966), some sarcomeres which had disintegrated and left behind debris which consisted of mitochondria, particles of glycogen and some filamentary structures. These changes were most common in the most peripheral sarcomeres, underneath the sarcolemmal membrane. They did not find any structural changes in the mitochondria, the sarcoplasmic reticulum, the sarcolemma or the nuclei, though the latter sometimes occurred in short chains or were in a central position in the fibre. Motor end-plates were found to be normal in the muscle biopsy of the patient studied by Godet-Guillain and Fardeau (1970).

Gustafsson and his colleagues in Stockholm (1965) conducted an electron microscope study of the muscles of rats made hypothyroid by means of radioactive iodine. They found a wider range than usual

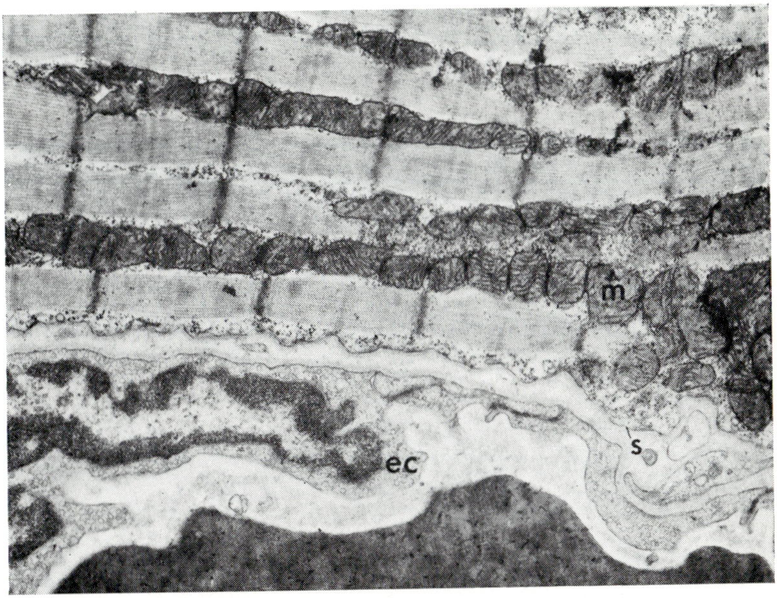

Figure 4.14(a). Same specimen as in Fig. 4.13, showing a peripheral part of a muscle fibre next to a blood vessel (ec). Note the cluster of mitochondria (M) underneath the sarcolemma (s). (×18,000). Compare with Fig. 4.14(b). (From Gustafsson *et al.*, 1965.)

of mitochondrial size in a few fibres, as well as an increased number of mitochondria which was most pronounced in the perinuclear region (Fig. 4.13) and beneath the sarcolemma in the vicinity of blood vessels (Fig. 4.14(a), (b)). In these regions they often found large numbers of tightly packed mitochondria. In neighbouring areas interfibrillar mitochondria frequently showed elongations which when joined together formed columns extending over a few sarcomeres (Fig. 4.15).

Gustafsson and his colleagues found that, generally speaking, the internal structure of the mitochondria did not differ from that of control animals, but that in areas where the mitochondria were enlarged, particularly in the interfibrillar region, there was an increase in the cristae relative to the matrix (Fig. 4.15). These long cristae were arranged in a rather parallel fashion, though less fre-

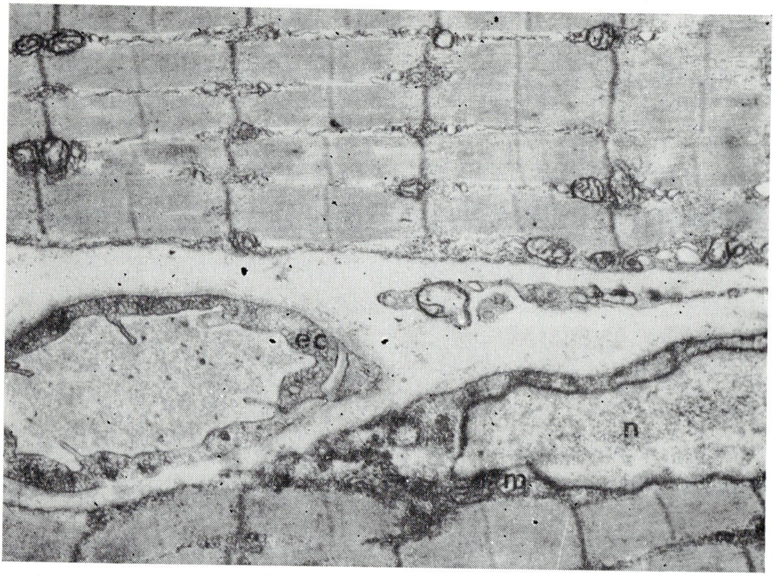

Figure 4.14(b). Longitudinal section of peripheral portions of two adjacent muscle fibres and transverse section of a blood vessel (ec) from the leg of a normal rat. Note the sparsely occurring mitochondria (M) in the subsarcolemmal regions of the two fibres and in the interfibrillar spaces of the upper fibre. A nucleus (N) is seen on the lower right. (From Gustafsson *et al.*, 1965.)

quently a honeycomb pattern was formed, which the authors thought was probably due to parallel, zig-zag cristae getting displaced. The sharp angles of the cristae seemed to anastomose, forming annular areas (Fig. 4.16). The mitochondrial apparatus overall in the muscles of these thyroidectomized rats was 1·5 times the size of that of controls.

It is difficult to know exactly what these ultrastructural changes signify, for in the patients of Norris and Panner (1966) and of

Bergouignan and his colleagues (1967) many of the changes persisted after thyroid hormone treatment had completely relieved the patients' symptoms. It seems likely from the studies of Spiro *et al.* (1970) that the severity and variety of the changes in the muscles of hypothyroid patients are a consequence of the great variation in the duration and degree of thyroid deficiency in different patients. Many of the pathological changes which have been described in

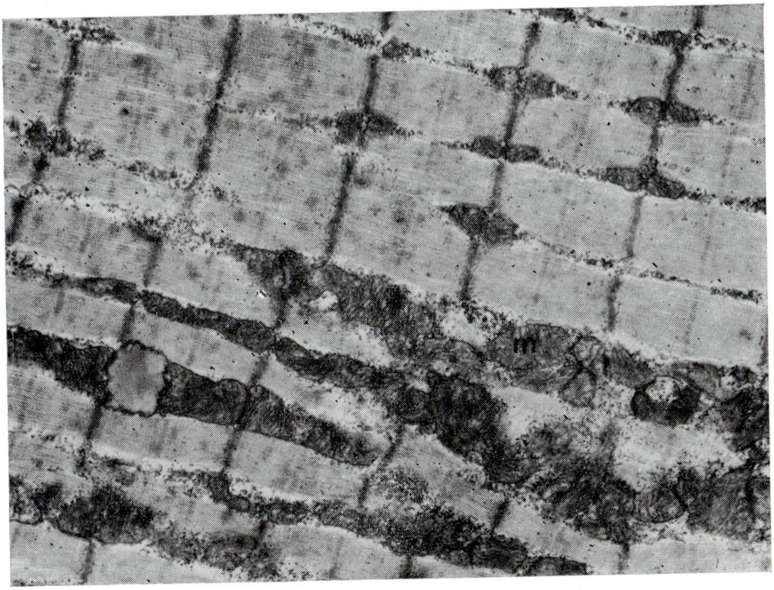

Figure 4.15. Longitudinal section through the central portion of a muscle fibre from a hypothyroid rat. Compared with Fig. 4.14(b) there are more interfibrillar mitochondria. In the lower left part of the figure there are some elongated mitochondria, averaging one sarcomere in length, some of which form columns running parallel to the fibre. Note the densely packed cristae. (×18,000). (From Gustafsson *et al.*, 1965.)

hypothyroid patients are not specific for that disease. Subsarcolemmal crescents have been found in other thyroid disease (Iversen, Asböe-Hansen and Carlsen, 1953). Dilatations in the sarcoplasmic reticulum have been found in both familial and thyrotoxic periodic paralysis (Engel, 1966), myotonic dystrophy (Schotland, 1968) and in muscular dystrophy (Pearce, 1966). Abnormal glycogen content is seen in other metabolic myopathies such as McArdle's syndrome (Schotland, Spiro and Rowland, 1965).

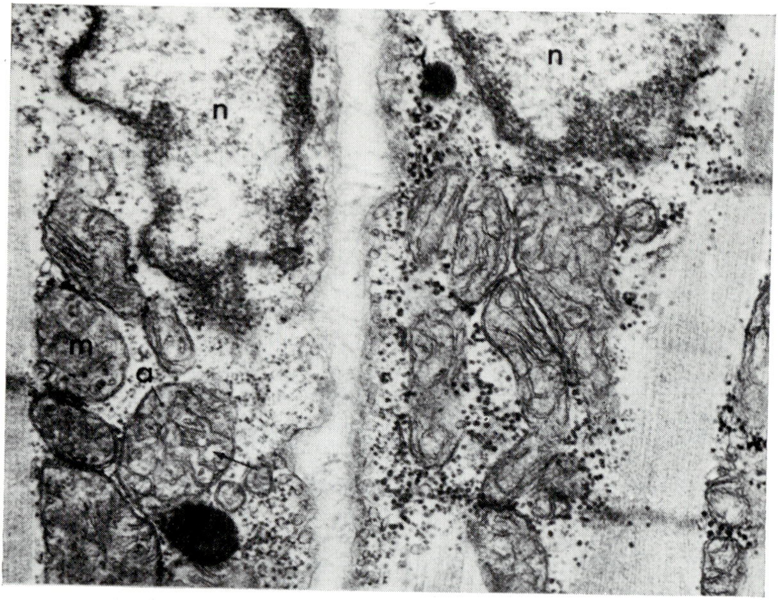

Figure 4.16. High power (×45,000) electron micrograph of same material as in Fig. 4.13. It shows a pattern of configuration of cristae which may be found in hypothyroid animals. Instead of being parallel the cristae tend to branch and join together forming a honeycomb pattern (arrow). Small annular structures (a) are seen in the matrix. (From Gustafsson *et al.*, 1965.)

Aetiology of hypothyroid myopathy

It has already been suggested (p. 128) that the muscle disorders of hypothyroidism belong to a continuous spectrum. At one end the patient with mild hypothyroidism presents with muscle aches and pains (Golding, 1970). The patient with more severe hypothyroidism gets muscle cramps and weakness of the proximal muscles and demonstrates myotonoid features with delayed muscle relaxation. Patients with the most severe forms of hypothyroidism may show muscle hypertrophy which could be partly due to an increase in individual muscle fibre diameter but also to the infiltration of the muscle by mucopolysaccharides. It is conceivable that this infiltration could have an effect on the physico-chemical characteristics of muscle and prevent normal relaxation (Thomasen, 1948; Nickel *et al.*, 1961). The electrically silent phenomenon of mounding or myoedema is also thought to be due to the infiltration. It is unlikely, however, that mucopolysaccharide infiltration is responsible for the weakness of hypothyroidism or the changes found on E.M.G., since mucopolysaccharide deposition does not occur in hypothyroidism secondary to pituitary disease (MacGregor, 1964) and myopathy has been found in at least two patients with this type of hypothyroidism (Aström, Kugelberg and Müller, 1961; Ramsay, 1971). In Ramsay's patient the symptoms developed while he was having cortisone replacement and did not disappear until six months after the introduction of thyroxine in adequate therapeutic dosage. In the patient of Aström, Kugelberg and Müller (1961), degenerative changes were found in the muscle fibres, but there was no evidence of infiltration by mucopolysaccharides. The patient had quite marked weakness of her muscles.

Although the temperatures of patients with hypothyroidism tend to be low and hypothermia has been shown to prolong Achilles reflex duration time (Waal-Manning. 1969), Lambert and his colleagues (1951) have shown that the slight decrease in muscle temperature is not sufficient to explain the prolongation found in hypothyroidism. Buchthal (1957) has also pointed out that cooling of the muscles tends to prolong mean action potential duration time, measured electromyographically, whereas shortened durations are usually found in hypothyroidism (p. 141). It seems likely therefore that any temperature change is of little or no importance in the muscle symptomatology of hypothyroidism.

Auto-immunity has been implicated in the aetiology of primary hypothyroidism (Roitt and Doniach, 1960) and recently Fakhri and Hobbs (1972) have shown a possible role of antibodies in the aetiology of exophthalmos. However, Fessel and Raas (1968) found no evidence that muscle auto-antibodies were present in their 4 hypothyroid patients with myopathy and since most patients make a full recovery after the institution of thyroid hormone therapy, it would seem unlikely that antibodies have anything to do with the muscle lesion.

One is left with the conclusion that the most important cause of hypothyroid myopathy is the effect of lack of thyroid hormone on the muscle fibre itself. Light microscopy does not suggest that a gross abnormality of muscle structure is responsible for the myopathy. However, electron microscopic studies reveal focal areas of myofibrillar degeneration and a varying incidence of mitochondrial structural change. These mitochondrial changes are not specific for hypothyroid myopathy since they have also been described in patients without thyroid disease (p. 153).

Gustafsson and his colleagues (1965) found that experimental hypothyroidism in rats brought about a marked hypertrophy and increase in the number of mitochondria. There was a decrease in mitochondrial respiration and phosphorylation relative to total mitochondrial protein or mass. Hoch (1967) has shown that the mitochondria of hypothyroid rats contain only 20% of the normal amount of thyroid hormone. The mitochondria respire too slowly and power is therefore decreased (Hoch, 1968). The thyroid hormone deficiency also, by virtue of its negative effect on protein synthesis (Tata *et al.*, 1963), causes a diminution of respiratory enzymes in the mitochondria. Mitochondria from hypothyroid rats contain reduced amounts of cytochrome b, c and $a + a_3$ (Maley, 1957; Kadenbach, 1966) and of flavoprotein catalysts (Rivlin and Langdon, 1966) compared with normal.

The net result of the deficiency of thyroid hormones on the mitochondria of skeletal muscle is a depressed production of ATP. Sarcotubular function may also be affected in hypothyroidism. Peter and his colleagues (1970) have shown a slow uptake of calcium by sarcotubular vesicles in hypothyroid rats. Since muscle contracts as a result of the calcium induced dephosphorylation of ATP, which causes activity of the cross-linkages between actin and myosin (Mommaerts, 1963; Price, 1969), the net result is muscle weakness. The muscles most affected in hypothyroidism are those which contain the most mitochondria, the proximal muscles (see p. 30). It is probable that these muscles, used largely for the maintenance of posture and for sustained effort, contain a preponderance of slow Type I fibres (Buchthal and Schmalbruch, 1970). Type I fibres have a greater abundance of mitochondria than fast, Type II fibres (Engel and Macdonald, 1970) and it is interesting that in the biopsy study of Spiro *et al.* (1970) the predominant atrophy in a cretin with myopathy was of the Type I fibres. After treatment the fibres returned to normal.

REFERENCES

Adams, R. D. (1969). In "Disorders of Voluntary Muscle". Edited by J. N. Walton, p. 157. Churchill, London.

Adams, R. D., Denny-Brown, D. and Pearson, C. M. (1962). In "Diseases of Muscle", pp. 231, 602. Kimpton, London.

Aikawa, J. K. (1956). The nature of myxedema; alterations in the serum electrolyte concentrations and radiosodium space and in the exchangeable sodium and potassium contents. *Ann. intern. Med.*, **44,** 30.

Arons, W. L., Vanderlinde, R. J. and Nusimovich, B. (1956). Exchangeable body sodium and potassium measurements in hyper- and hypothyroidism. *J. clin. Endocrinol.*, **16,** 974.

Asböe-Hansen, G., Iversen, K. and Wichmann, R. (1952). Malignant exophthalmos; muscular changes and thyrotropin content in serum. *Acta endocr.* (*Kbh.*), **11,** 376.

Aström, K.-E., Kugelberg, E. and Müller, R. (1961). Hypothyroid myopathy. *Arch. Neurol.*, **5,** 472.

Balls, K. F., Chamberlain, R. H., Rose, E., Gorson, R. O. and Blount, H. C. (1955). The treatment of thyrotoxicosis with radioiodine. *Radiology*, **64,** 858.

Bergouignan, M., Vital, C. and Bataille, J.-M. (1967). Les myopathies hypothyroïdiennes. Aspects cliniques et histopathologiques. *Presse Méd.*, **75,** 1551.

Berkheiser, S. W. (1955). Adult hypothyroidism: report of an advanced case with autopsy study. *J. clin. Endocrinol.*, **15,** 44.

Bowers, C. Y., Gordon, D. L. and Segaloff, A. (1959). The myxedema reflex in infants and children with hypothyroidism. *J. Pediat.*, **54,** 46.

Brewer, D. B. (1951). Myxoedema: an autopsy report with histochemical observations on the nature of the mucoid infiltrations. *J. Path. Bact.*, **63,** 503.

Buchthal, F. (1957). "Introduction to Electromyography," p. 16. p. 26, Glydendal, Copenhagen.

Buchthal, F. and Rosenfalck, P. (1963). Electrophysiological aspects of myopathy with particular reference to progressive muscular dystrophy. In "Muscular Dystrophy in Man and Animals". Edited by G. H. Bourne and M. N. Golarz, p. 193. Karger, Basel.

Buchthal, F. and Schmalbruch, H. (1970). Contraction times and fibre types in normal and diseased human muscle. In "Proceedings of an International Congress on Muscle Diseases, Milan, 1969". Edited by J. N. Walton, N. Canal and G. Scarlato, p. 131. Excerpta Medica, Amsterdam.

Chaney, W. C. (1924). Tendon reflexes in myxedema: a valuable aid in diagnosis. *J. Amer. med. Ass.*, **82,** 2013.

Cheek, D. B., Brasel, J. A., Elliott, D. and Scott, R. (1966). Muscle cell size and number in normal children and in dwarfs (pituitary, cretins and primordial) before and after treatment. *Bull. Johns. Hopk. Hosp.*, **119,** 46.

Collins, J. A. Jr., Zimmer, F. E., Johnson, W. J. and Kough, R. H. (1964). The many faces of hypothyroidism. *Postgrad. Med.*, **36,** 371.

Comings, D. E. (1962). Myxedema with Erb's limb girdle muscular dystrophy. Report of a case with a review of the muscular abnormalities of myxedema. *Arch. intern. Med.*, **109,** 724.

Crevasse, L. E. and Logue, R. B. (1959). Peripheral neuropathy in myxedema. *Ann. intern. Med.*, **50,** 1433.

Crispell, K. R. and Parson, W. (1954). The occurrence of myotonia in two patients following thyroidectomy for hyperthyroidism. In "Transactions of the American Goiter Association", p. 399. Thomas, Springfield, Illinois.

David, L., Bertrand, J., Pousset, G., Salle, B. and François, R. (1969). Thyroïdite d'Hashimoto et syndrome myopathique chez un enfant. *Lyon méd.*, **221,** 1493.

Debré, R. and Semelaigne, G. (1935). Syndrome of diffuse muscular hypertrophy in infants causing athletic appearance. Its connection with congenital myxedema. *Amer. J. Dis. Child.*, **50,** 1351.

Edelman, I. S., Olney, J. M., James, A. H., Brooks, L. and Moore, F. D. (1952). Body composition: studies in the human being by the dilution principle. *Science*, **115,** 447.

Ekbom, K., Hed, R., Herdenstam, C.-G. P. and Nygren, A. (1966). The serum creatine phosphokinase activity and the Achilles reflex in hyperthyroidism and hypothyroidism. *Acta med. scand.*, **179,** 433.

Engel, A. G. (1966). Electron microscopic observations in primary hypokalemic and thyrotoxic periodic paralyses. *Mayo Clin. Proc.*, **41,** 797.

Engel, A. G. (1970). Acid maltase deficiency in adults; studies in four cases of a syndrome which may mimic muscular dystrophy or other myopathies. *Brain*, **93,** 599.

Engel, A. G. and Gomez, M. R. (1970). Acid maltase levels in muscle in heterozygous acid maltase deficiency and in non-weak and neuromuscular disease controls. *J. Neurol. Neurosurg. Psychiat.*, **33,** 801.

Engel, A. G. and MacDonald, R. D. (1970). Ultrastructural reactions in muscle disease and thin light microscopic correlates. In "Proceedings of an International Congress in Muscle Diseases, Milan, 1969". Edited by J. N. Walton, N. Canal and G. Scarlato, p. 71. Excerpta Medica, Amsterdam.

Fakhri, O. and Hobbs, J. R. (1972). Detection of antibodies which can cooperate with lymphocytes. *Lancet*, *ii*, 403.

Fessel, W. J. (1968). Myopathy of hypothyroidism. *Ann. rheum. Dis.*, **27,** 590.

Fessel, W. J. and Raas, M. C. (1968). Autoimmunity in the pathogenesis of muscle disease. *Neurology* (*Minneap.*), **18,** 1137.

Fincham, R. W. and Cape, C. A. (1968). Neuropathy in myxedema. A study of sensory nerve conduction in the upper extremities. *Arch. neurol.*, **19,** 464.

Foster, M. and Barr, D. P. (1944). Myxedema; record of an autopsied case with special emphasis upon lesions of muscles. *J. clin. Endocrinol.*, **4,** 417.

Godet-Guillain, J. and Fardeau, M. (1970). Hypothyroid myopathy. Histological and ultrastructural study of an atrophic form. In "Proceedings of an International Congress on Muscle Diseases, Milan, 1969". Edited by J. N. Walton, N. Canal and G. Scarlato, p. 512. Excerpta Medica, Amsterdam.

Golding, D. N. (1970). Hypothyroidism presenting with musculoskeletal symptoms. *Ann. rheum. Dis.*, **29**, 10.

Graig, F. A. and Ross, G. (1963). Serum creatine-phosphokinase in thyroid disease. *Metabolism*, **12**, 57.

Graig, F. A. and Smith, J. C. (1965). Serum creatine phosphokinase activity in altered thyroid states. *J. clin. Endocrinol.*, **25**, 723.

Griffiths, P. D. (1965). Serum enzymes in diseases of the thyroid gland. *J. clin. Path.*, **18**, 660.

Gustafsson, R., Tata, J. R., Lindberg, O. and Ernster, L. (1965). The relationships between the structure and activity of rat skeletal muscle mitochondria after thyroidectomy and thyroid hormone treatment. *J. Cell. Biol.*, **26**, 555.

Harrell, G. T. and Daniel, D. (1941). Delayed relaxation of tendon reflexes as an aid in the diagnosis of myxedema. *North Carolina med. J.*, **2**, 549.

Hedley, A. J., Hall, R., Amos, J., Michie, W. and Crooks, J. (1971). Serum thyrotropin levels after subtotal thyroidectomy for Graves' disease. *Lancet*, *i*, 455.

Hess, J. W., MacDonald, R. P., Frederick, R. J., Jones, R. N., Neely, J. and Gross, D. (1964). Serum creatine phosphokinase activity in disorders of heart and skeletal muscle. *Ann. intern. Med.*, **61**, 1015.

Hesser, F. H. (1940). Hypertrophia musculorum vera (dystrophia musculorum hyperplastica) associated with hypothyroidism; a case study. *Bull. Johns Hopk. Hosp.*, **66**, 353.

Heuyer, G., Lebovici, S., Koupernik, C. and Martinetti, J. (1951). Hypertrophie musculaire du myxoedème congenital; effets du traitement. *Arch. franç. Pédiat.*, **8**, 557.

Hoch, F. L. (1967). Early action of injected L-thyroxine on mitochondrial oxidative phosphorylation. *Proc. nat. Acad. Sci.* (*Wash.*), **58**, 506.

Hoch, F. L. (1968). Biochemistry of hyperthyroidism and hypothyroidism. *Postgrad. med. J.*, **44**, 347.

Hoffmann, J. (1897). Weiterer Beitrag zur Lehre von der Tetanie. *Deutsch. Z. Nervenheilk*, **9**, 278.

Hurwitz, L. J., McCormick, D. and Allen, I. V. (1970). Reduced muscle α-glucosidase (acid maltase) activity in hypothyroid myopathy. *Lancet*, *i*, 67.

Iversen, K., Asböe-Hansen, G. and Carlsen, F. (1953). Electron microscopy of certain muscle lesions in patients with pituitary-thyroid disorders. *Acta endocr.*, (*Kbh.*) **14**, 177.

Kadenbach, B. (1966). The influence *in vivo* of thyroid hormones on oxidative phosphorylation and enzymic activities in mitochondria. *Biochem. Z.*, **344**, 49.

Kirchheiner, B. (1962). Specific muscle lesions in pituitary-thyroid disorders. *Acta med. scand.*, **172**, 539.

Kissel, P., Hartemann, P. and Duc, M. (1965). "Les Syndromes Myo-thyroïdiens." Masson, Paris.

Kleeman, C. R., Epstein, F. H., McKay, D. and Taborsky, E. (1958). Effects of hypo- and hyperthyroidism on the filterability of serum magnesium. *J. clin. Endocrinol. Metab.*, **18,** 1111.

Kobayashi, A. and Takeuchi, K. (1967). Magnesium levels and thyroid disease. *Lancet, ii,* 1152.

Kocher, T. (1892). Zur Verhütung des Cretinismus und cretinoider Zustände nach neuen Forschungen. *Dtsch. Z. Chir.*, **34,** 556.

Koster, J. F. (1970). Acid maltase activity and hypothyroidism. *Lancet, ii,* 1187.

Kriss, J. P., Pleshakov, V., Rosenblum, A. L., Holderness, M., Sharp, G. and Utiger, R. (1967). Studies on the pathogenesis of the ophthalmopathy of Graves' disease. *J. clin. Endocrinol. Metab.*, **27,** 582.

Kroll, A. J. and Kuwabara, T. (1966). Dysthyroid ocular myopathy. *Arch. Ophthal.*, **76,** 244.

Kugelberg, E. (1947). Electromyograms in muscular disorders. *J. Neurol. Neurosurg. Psychiat.*, **10,** 122.

Kugelberg, E. (1949). Electromyography in muscular dystrophies. Differentiation between dystrophies and chronic lower motor neurone lesions. *J. Neurol. Neurosurg. Psychiat.*, **12,** 129.

Kuhlbäck, B. (1957). Creatine and creatinine metabolism in thyrotoxicosis and hypothyroidism. A clinical study. *Acta med. scand.*, **159,** Suppl. 331.

Lambert, E. H., Underdahl, L. O., Beckett, S. and Mederos, L. O. (1951). A study of the ankle jerk in myxedema. *J. clin. Endocrinol.*, **11,** 1186.

Lambert, E. H. and Sayre, G. P. (1955). Myopathy in rabbits following thyroidectomy. *Amer. J. Physiol.*, **183,** 636.

Lapresle, J. and Fardeau, M. (1965). Diagnostic histologique des atrophies et hypertrophies musculaires. In "Proceedings, VIIIth International Congress of Neurology, Vienna, 1965", Vol. II, p. 47. Wiener Medizinische Akademie, Vienna.

Lawson, J. D. (1958). The free Achilles reflex in hypothyroidism and hyperthyroidism. *New Engl. J. Med.*, **259,** 761.

Lewitus, Z. and Bornstein, B. (1962). The mytonia-like syndrome of myxedema. *Israel med. J.*, **21,** 103.

Lieberthal, A. S., Benson, S. G. and Klitgaard, H. M. (1963). Serum malic dehydrogenase in thyroid disease. *J. clin. Endocrinol.*, **23,** 211.

Luft, R., Ikkos, D., Palmieri, G., Ernster, L. and Afzelius, B. (1962). A case of severe hypermetabolism of nonthyroid origin with a defect in the maintenance of mitochondrial respiratory control; a correlated clinical, biochemical and morphological study. *J. clin. Invest.*, **41,** 1776.

McCormick, D., Allen, I. V. and Hurwitz, L. J. (1971). Acid maltase activity and hypothyroidism. *Lancet, i,* 85.

MacGregor, A. G. (1964). Hypothyroidism, In "The Thyroid Gland", Vol. 2. Edited by R. Pitt-Rivers and W. R. Trotter, p. 120. Butterworths, London.

Maley, G. F. (1957). Comparison of some enzyme systems in normal and thyrotoxic rat livers. *Amer. J. Physiol.*, **188,** 35.

Mann, A. S. (1963). The value of kinemography in the diagnosis of thyroid dysfunction. *Amer. J. med. Sci.*, **245,** 317.

Marshall, R. J. and McCaughey, W. T. E. (1956). Hypothermic myxoedema coma with muscle damage and acute renal tubular necrosis *Lancet*, *ii*, 754.

Millikan, C. H. and Haines, S. F. (1953). The thyroid gland in relation to neuromuscular disease. *Arch. intern. Med.*, **92,** 5.

Mommaerts, W. F. H. M. (1963). The muscle cell and its functional architecture. *Amer. J. Med.*, **35,** 606.

Moosa, A. and Dubowitz, V. (1971). Slow nerve conduction velocity in cretins. *Arch. Dis. Child.*, **46,** 852.

Munro, D. S., Renschler, H. and Wilson, G. M. (1958). Exchangeable potassium and sodium in hyperthyroidism and hypothyroidism. *Metabolism*, **7,** 124.

Murray, I. P. C. and Simpson, J. A. (1958). Acroparaesthesia in myxoedema. A clinical and electromyographic study. *Lancet*, *i*, 1360.

Najjar, S. S. and Nachman, H. S. (1965). The Kocher-Debré-Semelaigne Syndrome. Hypothyroidism with muscular "hypertrophy". *J. Pediat.*, **66,** 901.

Nick, J. (1943). "Les atrophies myopathiques liées à l'insuffisance thyroïdenne acquise de l'adulte. Étude critique des syndromes myohypothyroïdiens de l'adulte." *Thèse. Méd., Paris.*

Nickel, S. N. and Frame, B. (1958). Neurologic manifestations of myxedema. *Neurology*, **8,** 511.

Nickel, S. N., Frame, B., Bebin, J., Tourtellotte, W. W., Parker, J. A. and Hughes, B. R. (1961). Myxedema neuropathy and myopathy. A clinical and pathologic study. *Neurology*, **11,** 125.

Norris, F. H. and Panner, B. J. (1966). Hypothyroid myopathy. Clinical, electromyographical and ultrastructural observations. *Arch. neurol.*, **14,** 574.

Ord, W. M. (1880). Cases of myxoedema. *Trans. clin. Soc., London*, **13,** 15.

Ozker, R. R., Schumacher, O. P. and Nelson, P. A. (1960). Electromyographic findings in adults with myxedema. Report of 16 cases. *Arch. phys. Med. Rehab.*, **41,** 299.

Pearce, G. W. (1966). Electron microscopy in the study of muscular dystrophy. *Ann. N.Y. Acad. Sci.*, **138,** 138.

Pearce, J. and Aziz, H. (1969). The neuromyopathy of hypothyroidism. Some new observations. *J. neurol. Sci.*, **9,** 243.

Pende, N. and Pende, V. (1952). L'atletismo mixedematoso. *Folia endocr.*, **5,** 133.

Peter, J. B., Worsfold, M. and Stempel, K. (1970). Mechanisms of hypermetabolism and of rapid contraction and relaxation of muscle in hyperthyroidism. In "Proceedings of an International Congress on Muscle Diseases, Milan, 1969". Edited by J. N. Walton, N. Canal and G. Scarlato, p. 506. Excerpta Medica, Amsterdam.

Pipberger, H., Kälin, R. and Wegmann, T. (1955). Muskuläre Störungen bei der Hypothyreose. *Schweiz. Med. Wschr.*, **85,** 420.

Poncher, H. G., Visscher, M. B. and Woodward, H. (1934). Creatinine metabolism in children with hypothyroidism. *J. Amer. med. Ass.*, **102,** 1132.

Poncher, H. G. and Woodward, H. (1936). Pathogenesis and treatment of myotonia congenita. *Amer. J. Dis. Child.*, **52,** 1065.

Price, H. M. (1969). In "Disorders of Voluntary Muscle". Edited by J. N. Walton, p. 29. Churchill, London.

Ramsay, I. D. (1971). Unpublished.

Ringqvist, I. (1970). Achilles reflex time as a measure of thyroid function. *Acta med. scand.*, **188,** 231.

Rivlin, R. S. and Langdon, R. G. (1966). Regulation of hepatic flavine adenine dinucleotide levels by thyroid hormone. *Advanc Enzyme Reg.*, **4,** 45.

Roitt, I. M. and Doniach, D. (1960). Thyroid auto-immunity. *Brit. med. Bull.*, **16,** 152.

Ross, G. T., Scholz, D. A., Lambert, E. H. and Geraci, J. E. (1958). Severe uterine bleeding and degenerative skeletal muscle changes in unrecognized myxedema. *J. clin. Endocrinol. Metab.*, **18,** 492.

Saito, M., Hibi, I., Kawazura, M. and Fukuyama, Y. (1963). Creatine-phosphokinase levels in hypothyroidism. *Lancet*, *ii*, 252.

Salick, A. I., Colachis, S. C. and Pearson, C. M. (1968). Myxedema myopathy: clinical, electrodiagnostic and pathologic findings in advanced case. *Arch. phys. Med.*, **49,** 230.

Schotland, D. L. (1968). Ultrastructural abnormalities in myotonic dystrophy including an unusual T system alteration. *J. Neuropath. exp. Neurol.*, **27,** 109.

Schotland, D. L., Spiro, D., Rowland, L. P. and Carmel, P. (1965). Ultrastructural studies of muscle in McArdle's disease. *J. Neuropath. exp. Neurol.*, **24,** 629.

Sharpe, A. R. (1961). A simple isotope method for recording the Achilles tendon reflex in myxedema. *J. Lab. clin. Med.*, **57,** 165.

Shorr, E., Richardson, H. B. and Mansfield, J. S. (1935). Influence of thyroid administration on creatin metabolism in myxedema of adults. *Proc. Soc. exper. Biol. Med.*, **32,** 1340.

Sjövall, K. and Voigt, A. (1964). Creatine-phospho-transferase isozymes. *Nature* (*Lond.*), **202,** 701.

Spiro, A. J., Hirano, A., Beilin, R. L. and Finkelstein, J. W. (1970). Cretinism with muscular hypertrophy (Kocher–Debré–Semelaigne Syndrome). Histochemical and ultrastructural study of skeletal muscle. *Arch. Neurol.*, **23,** 340.

Stanbury, J. B., Goldsmith, R. R. and Gillis, M. (1954). Myotonic dystrophy associated with thyroid disease. *J. clin. Endocrinol. Metab.*, **14,** 1437.

Tata, J. R., Ernster, L., Lindberg, O., Arrhenius, E., Pedersen, S. and Hedman, R. (1963). The action of thyroid hormones at the cell level. *Biochem. J.*, **86,** 408.

Thomasen, E. (1948). "Myotonia" (Opera ex Domo Biologiae Hereditarae Humanae Universitatis Hafniensis, Vol. 17), translated by FinnBrink Carlsen, Munksgaard, Copenhagen.

Thorn, G. W. (1936). Creatine studies in thyroid disorders. *Endocrinology*, **20,** 628.

Thorn, G. W. and Eder, H. A. (1946). Studies on chronic thyrotoxic myopathy. *Amer. J. Med.*, **1,** 583.

Waal-Manning, H. J. (1969). Effect of propanolol on the duration of the Achilles tendon reflex. *Clin. Pharmacol. Ther.*, **10,** 199.

Wade, A. F. (1957). A case of myotonia congenita with hypothyroidism. *Brit. med. J.*, *i*, 1223.

Waldstein, S. S., Bronsky, D., Shrifter, H. B. and Oester, Y. T. (1958). The electromyogram in myxedema. *Arch. intern. Med.*, **101,** 97.

Watson, E. M. and Pearce, R. H. (1947). Mucopolysaccharide content of the skin in localized (pre-tibial) myxedema. *Amer. J. clin. Path.*, **17,** 507.

Wayne, E. J. (1960). Clinical and metabolic studies in thyroid disease. *Brit. med. J.*, *i*, 78.

Weissbein, A. S. and Lawson, J. D. (1960). Paradoxical lengthening of muscle contraction time in hypothyroid patients given small doses of L-triiodothyronine, thyroxine and desiccated thyroid. *J. clin. Endocrinol. Metab.*, **20,** 429.

Weitz, W. (1931). Über eigentümliche Muskelerscheinungen bei Myxödem. *Deutsche Z. Nervenheilk*, **120,** 297.

Wilson, J. and Walton, J. N. (1959). Some muscular manifestations of hypothyroidism. *J. Neurol. Neurosurg. Psychiat.*, **22,** 320.

CHAPTER 5

THYROID FUNCTION IN MISCELLANEOUS MUSCLE DISORDERS

Myotonia congenita

Wade (1957) described a male hypothyroid patient aged 20 who had had myotonia congenita from the age of 5. Treatment with L-thyroxine improved the symptoms of myotonia but did not completely abolish them. There was evidence of myotonia also in the patient's mother, a maternal aunt and female cousin.

The patient reported by Jarcho and Tyler (1958) developed the symptoms of myotonia congenita about eight years before a partial thyroidectomy for multinodular goitre. Following the operation she developed hypothyroidism and the muscle symptoms were made much worse. They were greatly improved, but not abolished by thyroid hormone replacement. Myotonia congenita was found in the patient's two brothers and in one daughter.

In the cases reported by Wade (1957) and by Jarcho and Tyler (1958) there is no reason to believe that the association between hypothyroidism and mytonia congenita was anything other than fortuitous. It is probable that the symptoms of myotonia congenita were made worse because the pseudomyotonia of hypothyroidism (p. 128) was added to the already existing myotonia.

Myotonic dystrophy

A 36-year-old woman who had had hypothyroidism treated with thyroid extract since the age of 15 developed myotonic dystrophy (Stanbury, Goldsmith and Gillis, 1954). Neither the withdrawal of her thyroid medication nor its resumption seemed to make any difference clinically to her degree of myotonia.

Waring, Ravin and Walker (1940) found goitres in 3 out of the 13 patients with myotonic dystrophy which they studied. In the 7 patients in whom estimations of the basal metabolic rate (B.M.R.) were made, it ranged from −11 to −41%, with an average of −25%. However this was probably due to the reduction in muscle mass since cholesterol levels were normal and in one patient the administration of thyroid hormone made no difference to the myotonia.

Nodular goitres were found in 3 out of 8 patients studied by Jacobson, Schultz and Anderson (1955). They too, found that the B.M.R. was often reduced, with a mean level of -25%. However, the serum cholesterol and protein bound iodine levels and the uptake of radioactive iodine by the thyroid gland were all normal. Similar results have been obtained by Benda, Maletskos, Hutchinson and Thomas (1954). They concluded that myotonic dystrophy is frequently associated with a colloid goitre but that normal levels of circulating thyroid hormone are maintained. No abnormality in the turnover of thyroxine and triiodothyronine, the extrathyroidal thyroxine space, the thyroidal uptake of radioiodine, the radioiodine conversion ratio and the serum protein bound iodine was found in 4 patients with myotonic dystrophy by Kuhl, Halper and Dowben (1961), despite the low B.M.R. Once again there was no clinical improvement in the myotonia with thyroid replacement therapy.

Caughey and Brown (1950) claimed that 2 of their 9 patients with myotonic dystrophy had evidence of hypothyroidism. However, the diagnoses were only based on reduced B.M.R.s and raised serum cholesterol levels and can probably not be accepted as proven.

Muscular dystrophy

Although there is a tendency for the B.M.R. to be reduced in progressive muscular dystrophy (Tyler and Perkoff, 1951), the first case of the association of hypothyroidism and Erb's limb girdle muscular dystrophy was reported by Comings in 1962. Treatment with thyroid made no difference to the muscle weakness and it was concluded that the appearance of the two diseases in the same individual was co-incidental.

REFERENCES

Benda, C. E., Maletskos, C. J., Hutchinson, J. C. and Thomas, E. B. (1954). Studies of thyroid function in myotonia dystrophica. *Amer. J. med. Sci.*, **228,** 668.

Caughey, J. E. and Brown, J. (1950). Dystrophia myotonica: an endocrine study. *Quart. J. Med.*, **19,** 303.

Comings, D. E. (1962). Myxedema with Erb's limb girdle muscular dystrophy. *Arch. intern. Med.*, **109,** 724.

Jacobson, W. E., Schultz, A. L. and Anderson, J. (1955). Endocrine studies in 8 patients with dystrophia myotonica. *J. clin. Endocrinol.*, **15,** 801.

Jarcho, L. W. and Tyler, F. H. (1958). Myxedema, pseudomyotonia and myotonia congenita. *Arch. intern. Med.*, **102,** 357.

Kuhl, W. J., Halper, I. S. and Dowben, R. M. (1961). Thyroxine and tri-iodothyronine turnover studies in dystrophia myotonica. *J. clin. Endocrinol.*, **21,** 1592.

Stanbury, J. B., Goldsmith, R. R. and Gillis, M. (1954). Myotonic dystrophy associated with thyroid disease. *J. clin. Endocrinol.*, **14,** 1437.

Tyler, F. H. and Perkoff, G. T. (1951). Studies in disorders of muscle. VI. Is progressive muscular dystrophy an endocrine or metabolic disorder? *Arch. intern. Med.*, **88,** 175.

Wade, A. F. (1957). A case of myotonia congenita with hypothyroidism. *Brit. med. J.*, ***1*,** 1223.

Waring, J. J., Ravin, A. and Walker, C. E. (1940). Studies in dystrophia myotonica. II. Clinical features and treatment. *Arch. intern. Med.*, **65,** 763.

INDEX